Stahl's Illustrated

Alzheimer's Disease and Other Dementias

Stephen M. Stahl
University of California, San Diego

Debbi Ann Morrissette
Neuroscience Education Institute

Nancy Muntner
Illustrations

 CAMBRIDGE
UNIVERSITY PRES

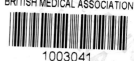

CAMBRIDGE
UNIVERSITY PRESS

University Printing House, Cambridge CB2 8BS, United Kingdom

Cambridge University Press is part of the University of Cambridge.

It furthers the University's mission by disseminating knowledge in the pursuit of education, learning and research at the highest international levels of excellence.

www.cambridge.org
Information on this title: www.cambridge.org/9781107688674

© Neuroscience Education Institute 2019

First published 2019

Printed in the United States of America by Sheridan Books, Inc.

A catalog record for this publication is available from the British Library

ISBN 978-1-107-68867-4 Paperback

This book is dedicated to...

Debbi Ann Morrissette's grandmother, Elizabeth Oleske, who suffered from Alzheimer's disease for over 20 years.

Dr. Stahl's father, Howard, who has suffered from Alzheimer's disease for many years.

And Dr. Morrissette's mother, Marie Henderson, the ultimate caregiver, who for nearly a decade opened her home and heart to countless individuals with dementia, and their families.

PREFACE

This book is designed to be fun, with all concepts illustrated by full-color images, figures, and tables supplemented by text. The visual learner will find that this book makes psychopharmacological concepts easier to master, and the non-visual learner may enjoy this book's short explanations of complex psychopharmacological concepts. Each chapter builds upon previous ones, synthesizing information about basic biology, diagnostics, treatment plans, complications, and comorbidities.

Novices may want to approach this book by first looking through all the graphics, gaining a feel for the visual vocabulary on which psychopharmacological concepts rely. After this once-over, we suggest going back through the book to read the text alongside the images. Learning from visual images and textual supplements should reinforce one another, providing novices with solid conceptual understanding at each step along the way.

Readers more familiar with these topics should find that going back and forth between the images and the text enables them to better understand complex psychopharmacological concepts. They may find themselves using this book frequently to refresh their psychopharmacological knowledge, and hopefully, they will refer their colleagues to this desk reference.

This book is intended as a conceptual overview of various topics. The authors provide you with a visual language to better understand the rules of psychopharmacology at the expense of discussing the exceptions to these rules. A References section at the back of this book gives you a good start for more in-depth learning about particular concepts.

Stahl's Essential Psychopharmacology (4th ed.) and *Stahl's Essential Psychopharmacology: The Prescriber's Guide* (6th ed.) can be helpful supplementary tools for more in-depth information on particular topics. You can also search the Neuroscience Education Institute's website (www.neiglobal.com) for articles, lectures, slides, and courses on psychopharmacological topics.

Whether you are a novice or an experienced psychopharmacologist, this book will hopefully lead you to think critically about the complexities of psychiatric disorders and their treatments.

Best wishes for your educational journey into the fascinating field of psychopharmacology!

Stephen M. Stahl

Table of Contents

CME Information

Release/Expiration Dates
Released: July, 2018
CME credit expires: June, 2021

Overview
The term "dementia" describes a collection of symptoms including cognitive dysfunction, memory loss, language and communication issues, and behavioral symptoms such as agitation. There are numerous causes of dementia ranging from neurodegenerative disorders to excessive alcohol use, and worldwide over 35 million individuals have some form of dementia. Alzheimer's disease is by far the most common cause of dementia, followed by vascular dementia and Lewy body dementia; however, many individuals present with pathological characteristics of more than one dementia (i.e., "mixed" dementia). Although dementia risk increases significantly with age, dementia is not necessarily an inevitable consequence of getting older. Furthermore, while many forms of dementia are irreversible (including Alzheimer's disease, frontotemporal lobar degeneration, and dementia with Lewy bodies), approximately 9% of individuals with dementia have potentially reversible conditions (e.g., vitamin deficiency, depression).

In this book, we will describe the most common causes of dementia, review best practices for differentially diagnosing dementia, as well as management strategies to help improve quality of life for both patients with dementia and the individuals who care for them.

Learning Objectives
After completing this activity, you should be better able to:

- Identify the neurobiological and molecular bases of Alzheimer's disease and other dementias

- Apply differential diagnostic assessment of patients with dementia according to established best practices

- Recognize the utility of currently available treatments for dementia

- Explore the state of research on novel compounds in development for the treatment of dementia

Accreditation and Credit Designation Statements

 Neuroscience Education Institute

The Neuroscience Education Institute (NEI) is accredited by the Accreditation Council for Continuing Medical Education (ACCME) to provide continuing medical education for physicians.

NEI designates this enduring material for a maximum of 8.0 *AMA PRA Category 1 Credits*™. Physicians should claim only the credit commensurate with the extent of their participation in the activity.

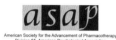
American Society for the Advancement of Pharmacotherapy
Division 55, American Psychological Association

The American Society for the Advancement of Pharmacotherapy (ASAP), Division 55 of the American Psychological Association, is approved by the American Psychological Association to sponsor continuing education for psychologists. ASAP maintains responsibility for this program and its content.

The American Society for the Advancement of Pharmacotherapy designates this program for 8.0 CE credits for psychologists.

Nurses and *Physician Assistants*: for all of your CE requirements for recertification, the ANCC and NCCPA will accept *AMA PRA Category 1 Credits*™ from organizations accredited by the ACCME. The content of this activity pertains to pharmacology and is worth 8.0 continuing education hours of pharmacotherapeutics.

Instructions for Optional Posttest and CME Credit

The estimated time for completion of this activity is 8.0 hours. There is a fee for the optional posttest (waived for NEI Members).

1. Read the book, evaluating the content presented

2. Complete the posttest, available only online at **www.neiglobal.com/CME** (under "Book")

3. Print your certificate (if a score of 70% or more is achieved)

Questions? Call 888-535-5600, or email CustomerService@neiglobal.com

Peer Review

This material has been peer-reviewed by a clinician specializing in dementia and Alzheimer's disease to ensure the scientific accuracy and medical relevance of information presented and its independence from commercial bias. NEI takes responsibility for the content, quality, and scientific integrity of this CME activity.

Disclosures

It is the policy of NEI to ensure balance, independence, objectivity, and scientific rigor in all its educational activities. Therefore, all individuals in a position to influence or control content are required to disclose any financial relationships. Although potential conflicts of interest are identified and resolved prior to the activity being presented, it remains for the participant to determine whether outside interests reflect a possible bias in either the exposition or the conclusions presented.

Disclosed financial relationships with conflicts of interest have been reviewed by the NEI CME Advisory Board Chair and resolved.

Author/Developer
Debbi A. Morrissette, PhD
Senior Medical Writer, Neuroscience Education Institute, Carlsbad, CA
No financial relationships to disclose.

Content Editor
Stephen M. Stahl, MD, PhD
Adjunct Professor, Department of Psychiatry, University of California, San Diego School of Medicine, La Jolla, CA
Honorary Visiting Senior Fellow, University of Cambridge, Cambridge, UK
Director of Psychopharmacology, California Department of State Hospitals, Sacramento, CA
Grant/Research: Acadia, Avanir, Braeburn, Intra-Cellular, Ironshore, Lilly, Neurocrine, Otsuka, Shire, Sunovion
Consultant/Advisor: Acadia, Adamas, Alkermes, Allergan, Arbor, Avanir, Axovant, ClearView, Concert, Ferring, Intra-Cellular, Janssen, Lilly, Lundbeck, Neos, Otsuka, Pfizer, Servier, Shire, Sunovion, Takeda, Taliaz, Teva, Tonix, ViroPharma
Speakers Bureau: Acadia, Lundbeck, Otsuka, Perrigo, Servier, Sunovion, Takeda
Board Member: Genomind

Peer Reviewer
Donna M. Wilcock, PhD
Sweeney-Nelms Professor, Alzheimer's Disease Research Center, Sanders-Brown Center on Aging, Department of Physiology, University of Kentucky College of Medicine, Lexington, KY
Speakers Bureau: AC Immune, Alector

The **Design Staff** has no financial relationships to disclose.

Disclosure of Off-Label Use
This educational activity may include discussion of unlabeled and/or investigational uses of agents that are not currently labeled for such use by the FDA. Please consult the product prescribing information for full disclosure of labeled uses.

Cultural and Linguistic Competency
A variety of resources addressing cultural and linguistic competency can be found at this link: nei.global/CMEregs

Provider
This activity is provided by NEI.
Additionally provided by the ASAP.

Support
This activity is supported solely by the provider, NEI.

Stahl's Illustrated | Objectives

- Identify the neurobiological and molecular bases of Alzheimer's disease and other dementias

- Apply differential diagnostic assessment of patients with dementia according to established best practices

- Recognize the utility of currently available treatments for dementia

- Explore the state of research on novel compounds in development for the treatment of dementia

The term "dementia" describes a collection of symptoms including cognitive dysfunction, memory loss, language and communication issues, and behavioral symptoms such as agitation. There are numerous causes of dementia ranging from neurodegenerative disorders to excessive alcohol use. Over 35 million individuals, worldwide, have some form of dementia. Alzheimer's disease is by far the most common cause of dementia, followed by vascular dementia and Lewy body dementia; however, many individuals present with pathological characteristics of more than one dementia (i.e., "mixed dementia").

Although dementia risk increases significantly with age, dementia is not necessarily an inevitable consequence of getting older. Furthermore, while many forms of dementia (including Alzheimer's disease, frontotemporal lobar degeneration, and dementia with Lewy bodies) are irreversible, approximately 9% of individuals with dementia have potentially reversible conditions (e.g., vitamin deficiency; depression).

In the following pages, we will describe the most common causes of dementia, review best practices for differentially diagnosing dementia, as well as management strategies to help improve quality of life for patients with dementia as well as the individuals who care for them. Chapters 1–4 describe the various types of dementia including their pathological and molecular substrates, which are often quite complex. We encourage all readers to refer to Chapter 5 (Treatment of Secondary Behavioral Symptoms of Dementia) for strategies to address the most common and often troublesome symptoms that are shared among many types of dementia (Alzheimer's Association, 2017; Maloney and Lahiri, 2016; Torrisi et al, 2017; Goodman et al, 2017).

Alzheimer's Disease

Although a disease-altering treatment has yet to be found, our understanding of Alzheimer's disease (AD) genetics and neurobiology has increased exponentially over the past few decades, as has our ability to detect Alzheimer's pathology using various biomarkers. In this chapter, we will review the genetic, pathological, and behavioral features of Alzheimer's disease and discuss how the use of biomarkers for the detection of AD has potentially opened up new avenues for the prevention (or possible reversal) of AD. Given the current absence of an effective pharmacological treatment, we will also describe how lifestyle may impact one's risk for developing AD and review potential strategies for reducing AD risk as well as reviewing currently available treatments aimed at ameliorating some of the symptoms of AD. For strategies to ameliorate some of the secondary behavioral symptoms often associated with Alzheimer's disease and other dementias, the reader is directed to Chapter 5.

The Cost of Alzheimer's Disease

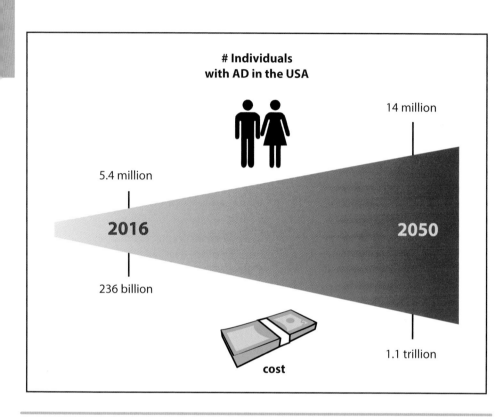

 # Individuals with AD in the USA

14 million

5.4 million

2016

2050

236 billion

1.1 trillion

cost

FIGURE 1.1. Alzheimer's disease (AD), the most common cause of dementia, is arguably the most devastating age-related disorder, with profound consequences to patients, family members, caregivers, and the economy. The latest data released by the Alzheimer's Association indicates that 5.4 million Americans presently have AD, costing the US approximately $236 billion annually. There is no cure for AD, and if no effective treatment is found by 2050, 14 million individuals will have AD—at an alarming annual cost of $1.1 trillion (Alzheimer's Association, 2017; Wimo et al, 2017).

Alzheimer's Disease Pathology

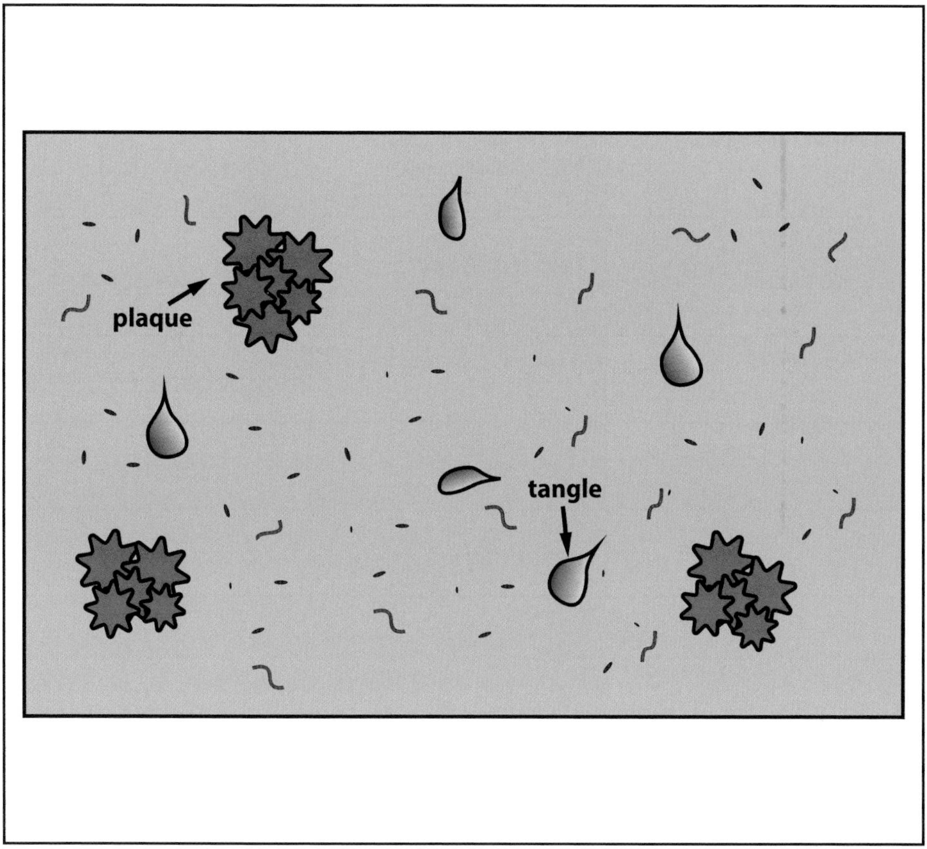

FIGURE 1.2. There are three major pathological hallmarks seen in the AD brain: plaques composed of the amyloid beta (Aβ) protein, neurofibrillary tangles (comprised of hyperphosphorylated tau protein), and substantial neuronal cell loss (Dugger and Dickson, 2017).

Progression of Alzheimer's Disease Pathology

Phase/Stage	Thal Phases of Amyloid Pathology	Braak Stages of Tau Pathology
1 and 2	neocortex and hippocampus	entorhinal cortices
3	striatum	hippocampus
4	brainstem	limbic cortices
5/6	cerebellum	neocortex

FIGURE 1.3. In the AD brain, Aβ and tau pathology and neurodegeneration typically progress according to slightly different patterns. In line with the Thal phases of amyloid progression, Aβ pathology usually presents first in the hippocampus and neocortex and progresses ultimately to brainstem and cerebellum. Conversely, tau pathology typically begins in the transentorhinal cortices and progresses (according to Braak staging) to multimodal association cortices. Neurodegeneration of the AD brain affects various areas that correlate with pathology including cortex, hippocampus, amygdala, basal forebrain, and brainstem. However, not all cases of AD (perhaps as many as 20%) have AD pathology that follows these typical pathological patterns (Dugger and Dickson, 2017; Hinz and Geschwind, 2017).

Amyloid Precursor Protein

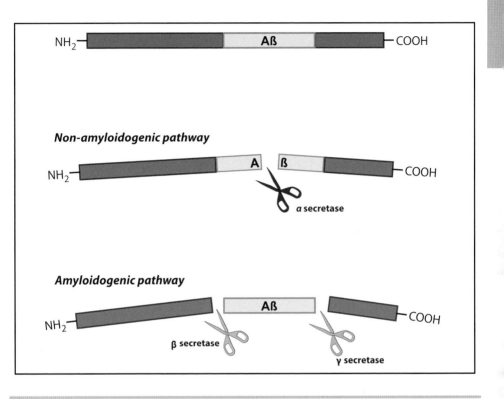

FIGURE 1.4. The Aβ protein is cut from a larger protein called the amyloid precursor protein (APP). There are two cleavage pathways by which APP may be processed: the non-amyloidogenic and the amyloidogenic pathways. In the non-amyloidogenic pathway, APP is cleaved by an enzyme termed β-secretase directly in the portion of APP where Aβ sits; processing of APP by β-secretase thereby precludes production of Aβ. In the amyloidogenic pathway, APP is first cleaved by β-secretase at the amino (NH$_2$) border of Aβ and then by β-secretase, an enzyme complex that includes presenilin as one of its main components. Mutations in the genes associated with AD (APP, PS1, and PS2) each lead to increased processing of APP via the amyloidogenic pathway. The discovery of these genes (and their effects on Aβ production) is arguably the main impetus behind the Amyloid Cascade Hypothesis (Arbor et al, 2016; MacLeod et al, 2015).

Amyloid Beta Isoforms

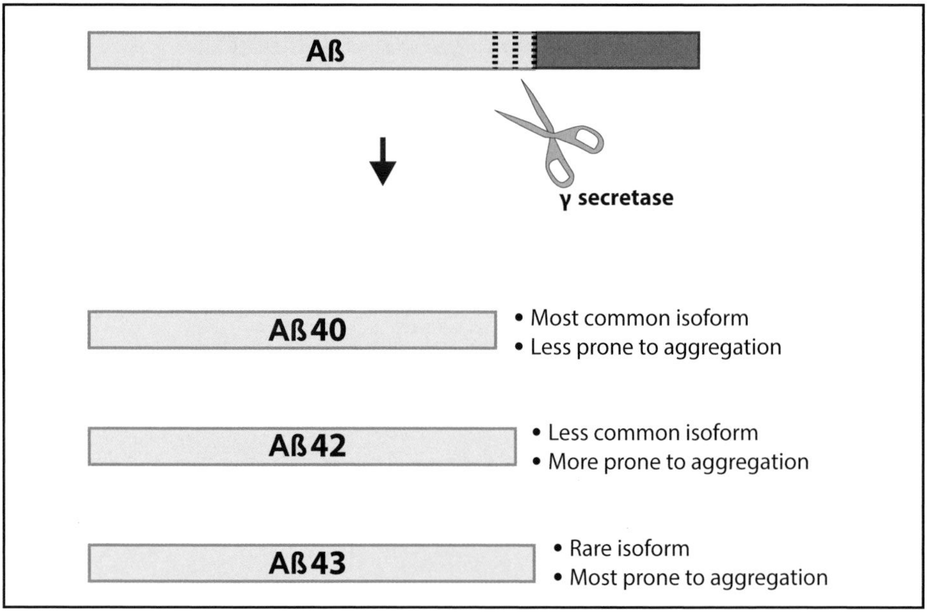

FIGURE 1.5. Gamma-secretase cleavage yields Aβ proteins ranging from 39 to 43 amino acids long. The Aβ40 isoform is the most common form; however, the Aβ42 isoform is more prone to aggregation into oligomers and is considered the more toxic form of Aβ. The Aβ43 isoform is relatively rare but is thought to be even more prone to aggregation than the Aβ42 isoform (Arbor et al, 2016; MacLeod et al, 2015).

Alzheimer's Disease Pathology: Amyloid Beta

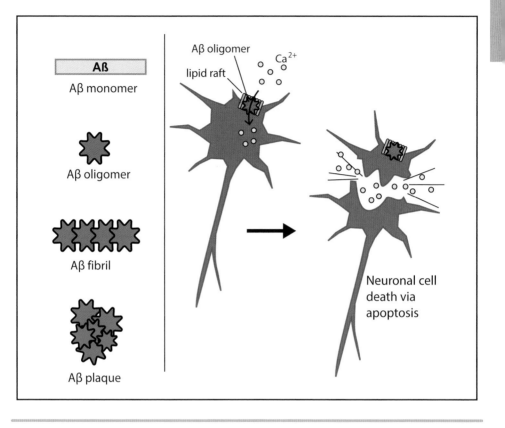

FIGURE 1.6. Although the accumulation of Aβ into plaques is a hallmark feature of AD, the most recent data indicate that it is the oligomeric form of Aβ (made from an accumulation of monomeric Aβ) and Aβ fibrils (formed by strings of Aβ oligomers) that may be the most toxic to the brain. One way in which Aβ oligomers may be toxic to neurons is via their effects on Ca^{2+} homeostasis within neurons. Aβ has been shown to form Ca^{2+} channels within the neuronal cell membrane, particularly in lipid raft domains. The resultant increase in Ca^{2+} influx via Aβ channels may ultimately lead to neuronal cell death via apoptosis (Arbor et al, 2016; MacLeod et al, 2015).

Is Amyloid Beta a Good Thing?

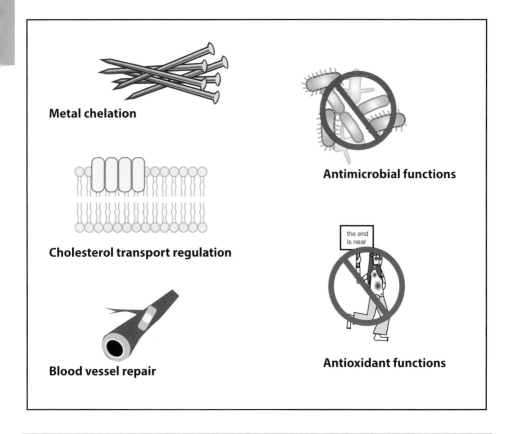

FIGURE 1.7. Although the production of Aβ has been historically associated with negative, pathological processes, it is a normal, healthy molecular process that we are only beginning to understand. Amyloid beta production has been hypothesized to have several potentially beneficial properties including chelation of metal ions; regulation of cholesterol transport; vessel repair; antimicrobial functions; and antioxidant activities, all of which may lend Aβ the ability to protect the brain as it ages, but may become pathologic under trying circumstances (Anand et al. 2012; Atwood et al, 2002; Atwood et al, 2002b; Kokjohn et al, 2012; Kumar et al, 2016; Cárdenas-Aguayo et al, 2014).

Alzheimer's Disease Pathology: Tangles

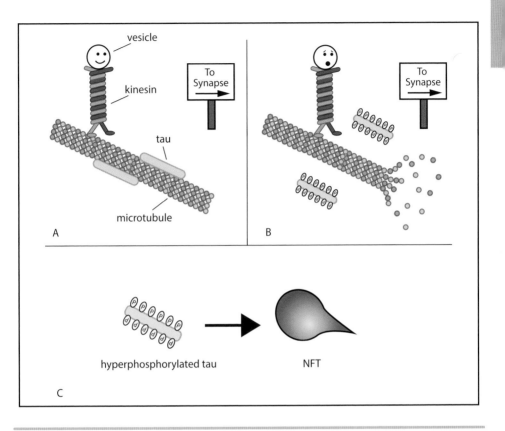

FIGURE 1.8. (A) Tau is a microtubule-associated binding protein and, in its non-pathological form, it binds to and stabilizes microtubules within axonal projections. It is along these microtubules that synaptic vesicles carrying neurotransmitters are transported to the synapse. (B) When hyperphosphorylated tau (pTau) is no longer able to bind microtubules, destabilization of microtubules and synaptic dysfunction results. (C) Hyperphosphorylated tau also forms paired helical filaments which then aggregate into the neurofibrillary tangles (NFTs) observable in the postmortem AD brain (Arendt et al, 2016).

Tauopathies

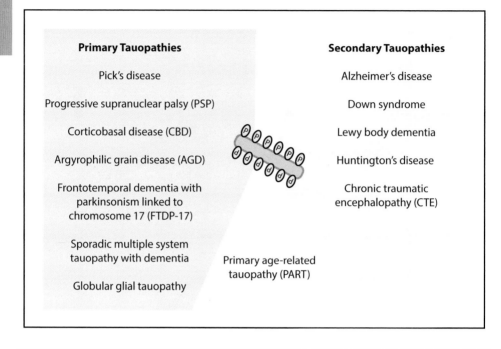

Primary Tauopathies

Pick's disease

Progressive supranuclear palsy (PSP)

Corticobasal disease (CBD)

Argyrophilic grain disease (AGD)

Frontotemporal dementia with parkinsonism linked to chromosome 17 (FTDP-17)

Sporadic multiple system tauopathy with dementia

Globular glial tauopathy

Primary age-related tauopathy (PART)

Secondary Tauopathies

Alzheimer's disease

Down syndrome

Lewy body dementia

Huntington's disease

Chronic traumatic encephalopathy (CTE)

FIGURE 1.9. Alzheimer's disease is only one type of dementia in which there is a pathological build-up of tau protein (i.e., AD is only one type of tauopathy). There are other tauopathies, some considered "primary" (tau is thought to be the driving pathological entity) and others, such as AD, considered "secondary" (a pathological entity other than tau is considered to be the driving force) (Arendt et al, 2016). Interestingly, there are some elderly individuals who exhibit only tau pathology (termed primary age-related tauopathy or PART); such individuals typically do not exhibit severe cognitive deficits or dementia. Thus, one might suppose that it is not tau (nor Aβ) accumulation that brings about dementia, but a cumulative process in which Aβ and tau may be the resultant features (Dugger and Dickson, 2017; Maloney and Lahiri, 2016).

Alzheimer's Disease Pathology: Neuronal Death

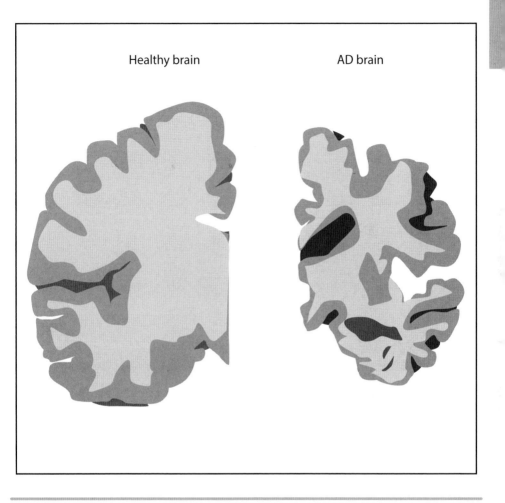

Healthy brain   AD brain

FIGURE 1.10. The loss of neurons is often so profound that it can be seen upon postmortem gross examination of the brain. Loss of neurons occurs in limbic and cortical regions and profoundly affects cholinergic neurons, although other neurotransmitter systems are also impacted. Neuronal cell death in AD is hypothesized to arise from several different factors including toxic oligomeric forms of Aβ, accumulated tau proteins, oxidative stress, and excitotoxicity (Pepeu and Giovannini, 2017; Alzheimer's Association, 2017).

Inflammation in Alzheimer's Disease

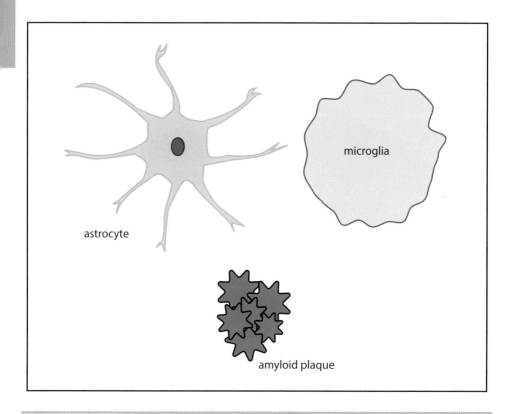

FIGURE 1.11. In the AD brain, Aβ plaques and NFTs are often surrounded by activated microglia and astrocytes, the brain's primary defense cells, indicating a substantial immune reaction in the AD brain. Many researchers hypothesize that Aβ (and possibly tau) set off an immune response in the brain that is intended to protect neurons from pathological entities. However, as the accumulation of pathological Aβ and tau levels increase, the brain's immune system becomes overwhelmed and inflammatory processes (including the release of cytokines and other inflammatory molecules) lead to the initial immune reaction, causing more harm than benefit to the brain. Proinflammatory factors may also increase amyloidogenic processing of APP, bringing about increased production of Aβ42 as well as hyperphosphorylation of tau (Bronzuoli et al, 2016; Ransohoff, 2016; Schwartz and Deczkowska, 2016).

The Amyloid Cascade Hypothesis

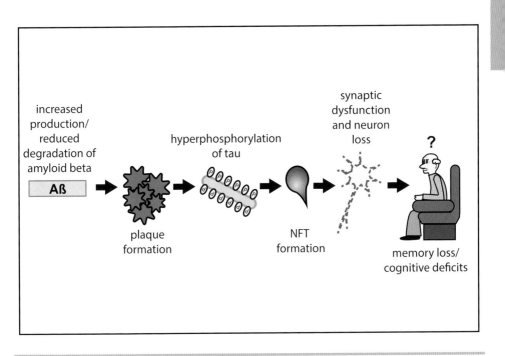

FIGURE 1.12. The leading hypothesis regarding the neurobiological progression of AD—the Amyloid Cascade Hypothesis—posits that the Aβ protein begins to accumulate in the brain with age due either to increased production or decreased degradation of Aβ and as a result of genetic and/or environmental factors. As Aβ accumulates, it also causes activation of several kinases (including glycogen synthase kinase 3β [GSK-3β], cAMP-dependent protein kinase [PKA], and cyclin-dependent protein kinase 5 [CDK-5]); these kinases cause hyperphosphorylation of tau. As AD progresses, synaptic dysfunction spreads, neurons are destroyed, and clinical signs of AD become increasingly severe (Mendiola-Precoma et al, 2016; Stahl, 2013).

Is The Amyloid Cascade Hypothesis Correct?

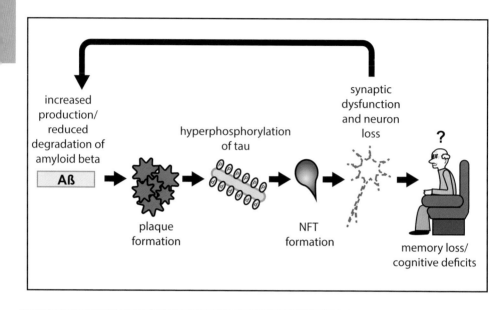

FIGURE 1.13. Not all experts are convinced that the Amyloid Cascade Hypothesis is correct, especially given the failure of all clinical trials utilizing treatments that target Aβ in patients with AD. However, proponents of the Amyloid Cascade Hypothesis claim that previous anti-amyloid clinical trials have failed not because the Amyloid Cascade Hypothesis is wrong, but because the subjects enrolled in such trials have been too far progressed in terms of the irreversible damage to the brain. All previously failed trials have enrolled patients with, at worst, clinically diagnosable AD or, at best, mild cognitive impairment (MCI), the clinical precursor to AD. Many Amyloid Cascade Hypothesis supporters theorize that once the amyloid cascade is set into motion, the detrimental effects (including oxidative stress, inflammation, the formation of neurofibrillary tangles [NFTs], and synaptic dysfunction) become a self-perpetuating cycle of destruction whereby Aβ accumulation becomes irrelevant. Accordingly, it is thought that anti-amyloid therapies must be initiated at the earliest sign of Aβ accumulation possible—before the amyloid cascade is irreversibly set into motion (and consequently before clinical signs of AD or even MCI are evident) (Alzheimer's Association, 2017; Arendt et al, 2016; Harrison and Owen, 2016).

Interaction of Aβ and Tau

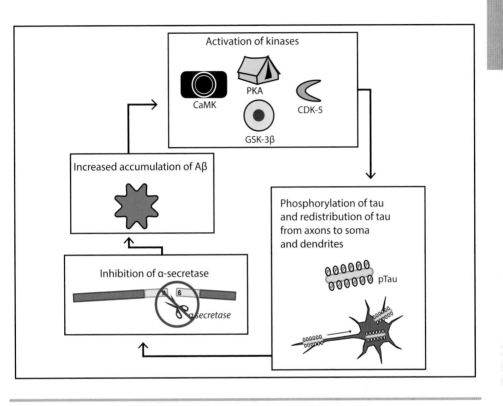

FIGURE 1.14. Most data support the hypothesis that Aβ sparks the hyperphosphorylation of tau in the AD brain. Not only may Aβ activate kinases such as glycogen synthase kinase-3β (GSK-3β), cyclin-dependent kinase-5 (CDK-5), cAMP-dependent protein kinase (PKA), and Ca^{2+}/calmodulin-dependent protein kinase-II (CaMKII) that phosphorylate tau, oligomeric Aβ, in particular, may also cause the redistribution of tau from axons to neuronal soma and dendrites, further disrupting neuronal function. There is also evidence that hyperphosphorylated tau (pTau) may actively drive Aβ pathology as well. One proposed mechanism for this is the pTau-induced inhibition of non-amyloidogenic (i.e., β-secretase) processing of amyloid precursor protein (APP). Thus, once the cascade of events initiated by Aβ has begun, a self-perpetuating cycle of pathological feedback is maintained (Arendt et al, 2016).

Familial Alzheimer's Disease

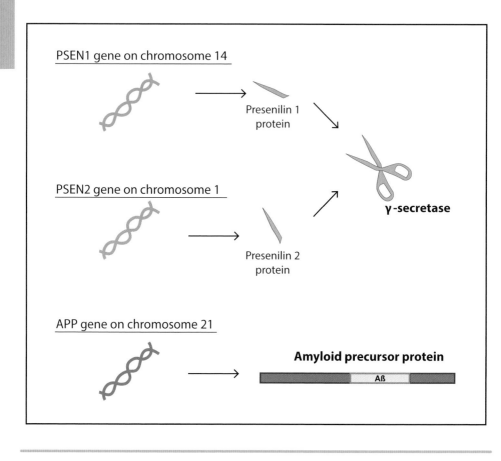

FIGURE 1.15. A small portion (~1%) of AD cases are familial—caused by mutations in one of three genes (presenilin 1 [PSEN1], presenilin 2 [PSEN2], or amyloid precursor protein [APP]). Amyloid beta (Aβ), a pathological protein that accumulates in AD, is cleaved from APP by β-secretase, an enzyme complex that contains presenilins. Inheritance of a mutation in any one of these genes leads to an increase in the production or pathogenicity of Aβ and the inevitable development of clinically diagnosable AD, typically before the age of 65 (Giri et al, 2016; Hinz and Geschwind, 2017).

Amyloid Precursor Protein Mutations

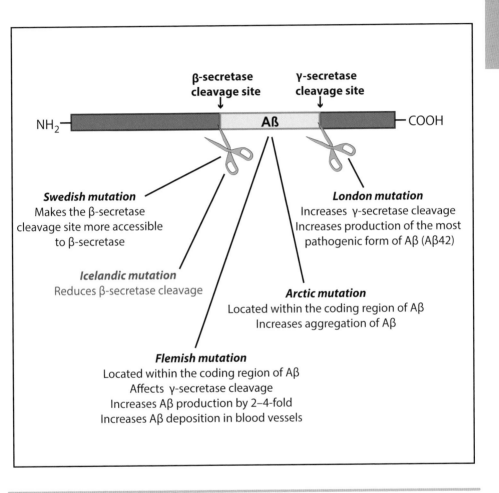

FIGURE 1.16. There are nearly 300 different AD-related mutations that have so far been discovered in the APP gene (including the Swedish, Arctic, London, and Flemish mutations) that are associated with familial AD. Most of these mutations can be found within or near the sites where Aβ is cleaved from APP (i.e., beta- and gamma-secretase cleavage sites). Another mutation, the Icelandic, has recently been discovered; individuals with the Icelandic mutation in APP appear to be protected from the development of AD (Giri et al, 2016; Hinz and Geschwind, 2017; Rosenberg et al, 2016; Schellenberg and Montine, 2012).

Presenilin Mutations

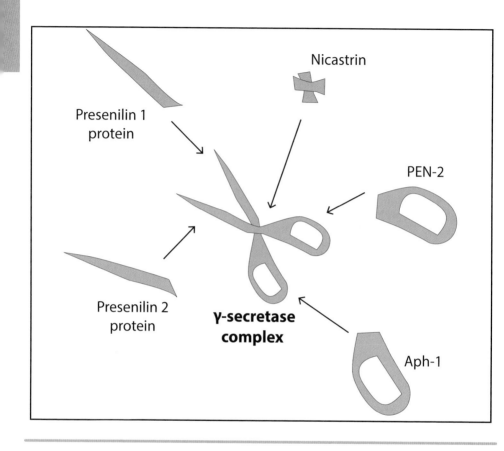

FIGURE 1.17. The PSEN1 and PSEN2 genes code for presenilins, which are active portions of the γ-secretase enzyme that cleaves APP (along with nicastrin, anterior pharynx-defective-1 [Aph-1], and presenilin-enhancer-2 [PEN-2]. There are 215 AD-related mutations in PSEN1 that have been discovered to-date, and these PSEN1 mutations account for approximately 50% of all familial, early-onset cases of AD; mutations in PSEN2 (of which 13 have so far been revealed) are far less common. Both PSEN1 and PSEN2 mutations lead to increased production of the more toxic Aβ42 protein, with the effects of PSEN1 mutations being more severe than those associated with PSEN2 mutations (Giri et al, 2016; Hinz and Geschwind, 2017).

Down Syndrome

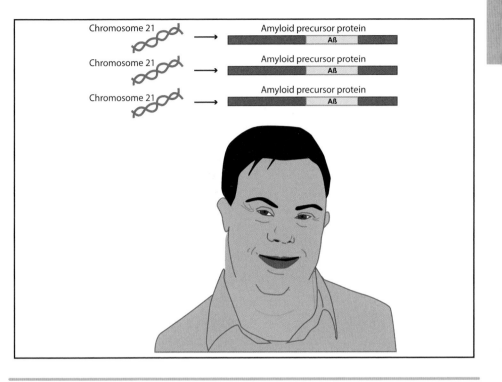

FIGURE 1.18. Individuals with Down syndrome have three copies of chromosome 21 (trisomy 21), thus they have three copies of the APP gene (individuals without trisomy 21 have only two copies). Due to the extra copy of the APP gene, individuals with Down syndrome produce excess APP protein and consequently have increased production and accumulation of Aβ. As a result, most individuals with Down syndrome have Alzheimer's pathology present in the brain by age 40, and most individuals with Down syndrome over the age of 70 exhibit Alzheimer's-type dementia (Ballard et al, 2016; Hithersay et al, 2017).

Sporadic Alzheimer's Disease

Increased Risk	Decreased Risk
Head injury	Cognitive stimulation
African–American race	Exercise
Depression	Mediterranean diet
Cardiovascular disease	Increased education
Diabetes	Social engagement
APOEε4 allele	APP Icelandic mutation
Additional genetic factors	Additional genetic factors

FIGURE 1.19. The vast majority of AD cases are sporadic—caused not by a single genetic polymorphism but by the combination of a plethora of identified and unidentified genetic and environmental factors (including apolipoprotein 4 [APOE4] allele status, education level, and cardiometabolic factors). Likewise, there are several environmental and lifestyle factors that appear to convey some protection against the development of AD, such as social engagement and exercise (Alzheimer's Association, 2017; Jonsson et al, 2012; Hardman et al, 2016; Larson et al, 2006; Lee et al, 2016; Michel, 2016; Uzun et al, 2011; Yaffe et al, 2012).

Alzheimer's Disease Risk Genes

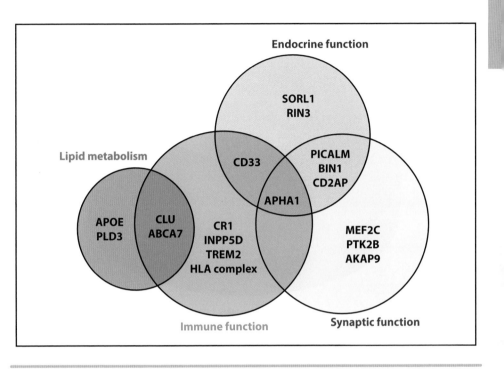

FIGURE 1.20. Numerous genetic polymorphisms have been indicated as increasing one's risk of developing AD. These genes largely fall into four categories in terms of their function: immunity, synaptic function, endocytosis, and lipid metabolism. Although inheritance of any one of these polymorphisms will not invariably lead to the development of AD, inheritance of several of these polymorphisms (in combination with environmental and other genetic factors) is hypothesized to accumulate into an increased risk of developing AD (Hinz and Geschwind, 2017).

ABCA7: ATP binding cassette subfamily A member 7; AKAP9: A-kinase anchoring protein 9; APHA1: aminoglycoside phosphotransferase A1; APOE: apolipoprotein E; BIN1: bridging integrator 1; CD2AP: cluster of differentiation 2-associated protein; CD33: cluster of differentiation 33; CLU: clusterin; MEF2C: myocyte enhancer factor 2C; PICALM: phosphatidylinositol-binding clathrin assembly protein; PLD3: phospholipase D family member 3; PTK2β: protein tyrosine kinase 2 beta; RIN3: renin angiotensin system (Ras) and Ras-associated binding protein (Rab) interactor 3; SORL1: sortilin-related receptor 1

Apolipoprotein E

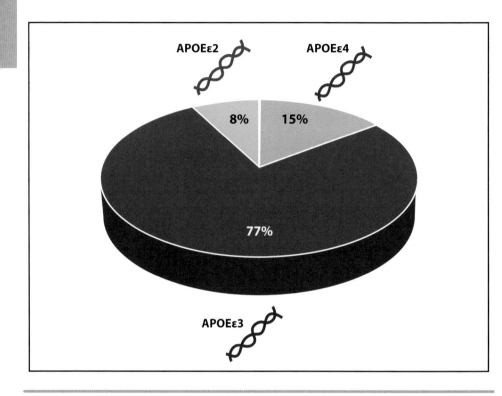

FIGURE 1.21. Of the genetic factors that contribute to the risk of developing AD, the gene for apolipoprotein E (APOE) appears to have the greatest influence. APOE is a protein that transports the cholesterol needed by neurons for synapse development, dendrite formation, long-term potentiation, and axonal guidance. APOE is also hypothesized to have an intricate relationship with amyloid beta (Aβ) whereby it may affect Aβ metabolism, aggregation, and deposition in the brain. Inheritance of even one copy of the APOEY4 allele increases the risk of developing AD by 3×; inheritance of two copies of APOEY4 increases the AD risk by 10×. Conversely, the APOEY2 allele appears to offer some protection from AD whereas the APOEY3 allele (the most common form of the APOE gene) conveys a risk that falls between APOEY2 and APOEY4. Approximately 15% of individuals in the general population carry the APOEY4 allele; however, among individuals with AD, 44% carry the APOEY4 allele (Alzheimer's Association, 2017; Arbor et al, 2016; Deypere et al, 2016; Giri et al, 2016; Hinz and Geschwind, 2017; Maloney and Lahiri, 2016).

Cholesterol and Alzheimer's Disease

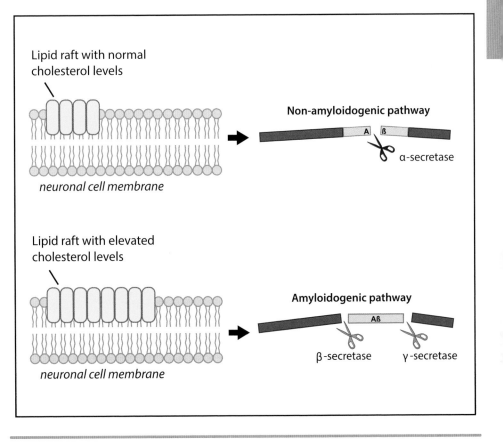

FIGURE 1.22. The brain contains 20% of the body's cholesterol, primarily in myelin sheaths and also, importantly, in lipid rafts. Lipid rafts are areas of the cell membrane that are critical for protein movement into and out of neurons, signal transduction, and neurotransmission. Of interest, Y-secretase cleavage of APP occurs within lipid rafts and, as aforementioned, Aβ oligomers are capable of forming Ca^{2+} channels within lipid rafts. Alterations in brain cholesterol levels have been shown to modify APP metabolism whereby ideal brain cholesterol levels may promote non-amyloidogenic (Y-secretase) processing of APP (and lower Aβ production) whereas elevated brain cholesterol levels may increase amyloidogenic (β- and Y-secretase) processing of APP (and consequently increase Aβ production) (Arbor et al, 2016; Mendiola-Precoma et al, 2016).

Type 3 Diabetes?

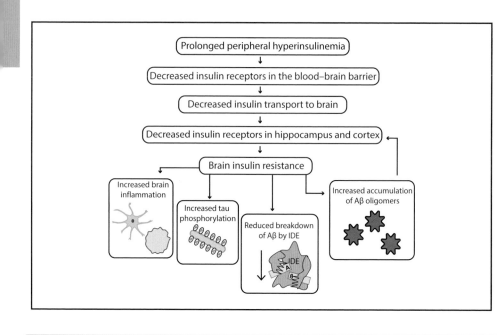

FIGURE 1.23. Individuals with Type 2 diabetes have a 2× greater risk of developing AD. In fact, it has been proposed that AD might represent a "Type 3" diabetes. Patients with AD not only show decreased insulin sensitivity in the periphery and a higher rate of Type 2 diabetes but also have increased insulin resistance and decreased insulin receptor expression within the brain, as well as decreased insulin transport into the brain. These insulin abnormalities are most notable in the medial temporal lobe—an area greatly affected in AD—and may be exacerbated by Aβ accumulation. Additionally, insulin degrading enzyme (IDE) not only breaks down insulin but also Aβ; with decreased insulin levels in the brain, there is a concomitant decrease in IDE levels. Given the association of Type 2 diabetes with obesity, the AD-as-Type-3-diabetes hypothesis may be one way in which certain lifestyle factors (e.g., high fat diet, low exercise) may increase one's risk of developing AD. In addition to modification of lifestyle factors that are beneficial in managing or preventing AD, intranasal delivery of insulin (providing a direct route to the brain) shows some promise in improving cognition and potentially decreasing AD risk (Chakraborty et al, 2017; Kullmann et al, 2016; Lee et al, 2016; Zillox et al, 2016).

Nutrition and Alzheimer's Disease

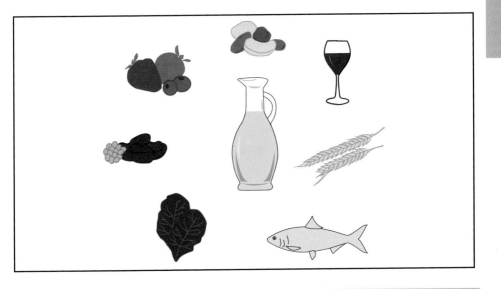

FIGURE 1.24. Numerous nutritional factors have been found to potentially lower one's risk, or slow the onset, of cognitive decline and dementia. Among these are long-chain omega-3 fatty acids (including monounsaturated fatty acids [MUFAs] found in olive oil and polyunsaturated fatty acids [PUFAs] such as eicosapentaenoic acid [EPA] and docosahexaenoic acid [DHA] from fish); vitamins C, E, and B12; folate; flavonoids; phenols; and carotenes. One particular diet found to contain such nutrients is the Mediterranean diet (MeDi); the MeDi includes green, leafy vegetables; nuts; berries; legumes; whole grains; abundant consumption of extra virgin olive oil; regular consumption of fish; and a modest (but consistent) intake of wine; red meat and dairy products are consumed only in very limited quantities. Conversely, diets that are high in saturated fats and refined carbohydrates may add to one's risk of developing AD. Not only has the Mediterranean diet been shown to improve cardiovascular health and reduce the risk for cancer; to-date, several preclinical and epidemiological studies have shown that adherence to the Mediterranean diet may also reduce age-related brain atrophy, improve cognition (including memory), slow cognitive decline, and possibly reduce one's risk of developing dementia (Anastasiou et al, 2017; Aridi et al, 2017; Cederholm, 2017; Gu et al, 2015; Hardman et al, 2016; Knight et al, 2016; Marcason, 2015; Lim et al, 2016; Petersson and Philippou, 2016; O'Donnell et al, 2015).

The Mediterranean Diet: Extra-Virgin Olive Oil

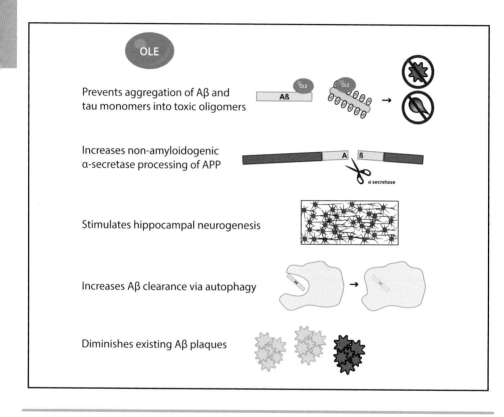

FIGURE 1.25. Accumulating data suggest that phenolic compounds (including oleuropein aglycone [OLE] and oleocanthal [OLC]), which are most notably found in extra-virgin olive oil (a staple of the Mediterranean diet), can actually thwart the pathological processes involved in Alzheimer's disease progression. Emerging data show that OLE prevents aggregation of both Aβ and tau, stimulates non-amyloidogenic processing of APP, enhances hippocampal neurogenesis, and increases clearance of Aβ (Rigacci, 2015; Qosa et al, 2015).

The Mediterranean Diet:
Extra-Virgin Olive Oil

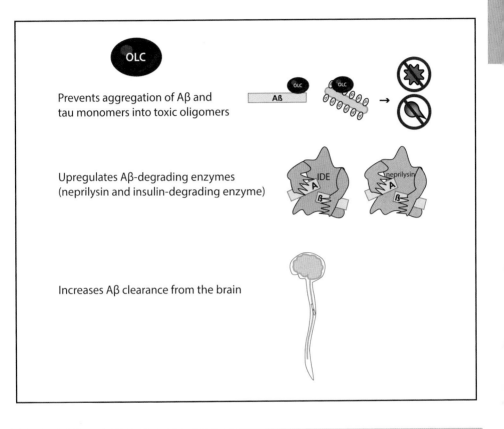

FIGURE 1.26. Similar to OLE, oleocanthal (OLC), another phenolic compound found in extra-virgin olive oil, has been shown to prevent aggregation of both Aβ and tau, as well as increasing breakdown and clearance of Aβ (Rigacci, 2015; Qosa et al, 2015).

The FINGER Trial

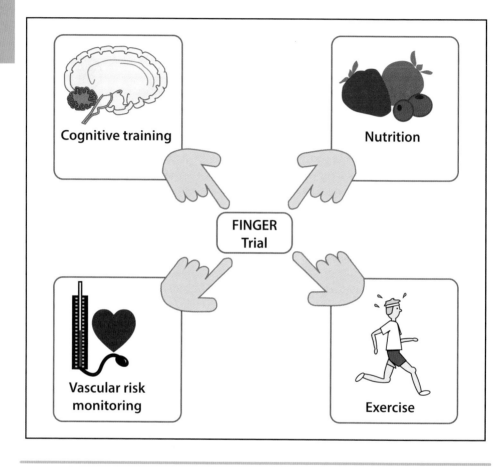

FIGURE 1.27. Recent efforts by researchers striving to test whether a multi-domain approach, involving small adjustments in several modifiable risk factors during pre-dementia phases in at-risk individuals, may halt or slow cognitive decline, and potentially dementia, are currently underway. The Finnish Geriatric Intervention Study to Prevent Cognitive Impairment and Disability (FINGER) and US Study to Protect Brain Health Through Lifestyle Intervention to Reduce Risk (US POINTER) are two such ongoing trials with promising preliminary results (Ngandu et al, 2015).

Hearing Loss in Alzheimer's Disease: Common Cause Hypothesis

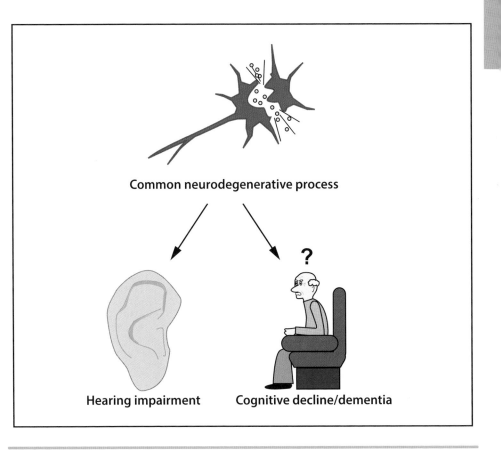

FIGURE 1.28. Hearing loss is associated with neurodegeneration and may lead to cognitive decline and increase one's risk of developing dementia. Three mechanisms by which hearing loss increases the risk of dementia have been proposed. The Common Cause Hypothesis posits that both hearing loss and cognitive decline are due to the same neurodegenerative process (Stahl, 2017).

Hearing Loss in Alzheimer's Disease: Cascade Hypothesis

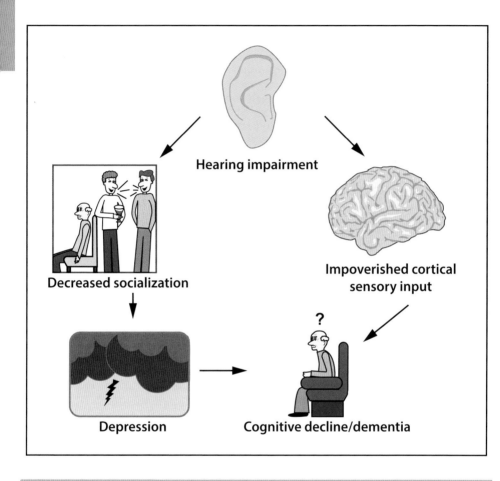

FIGURE 1.29. The Cascade Hypothesis proposes that auditory deprivation leads to cognitive decline via decreased socialization, depression, and reduced sensory input (Stahl, 2017).

Hearing Loss in Alzheimer's Disease: Cognitive Load Hypothesis

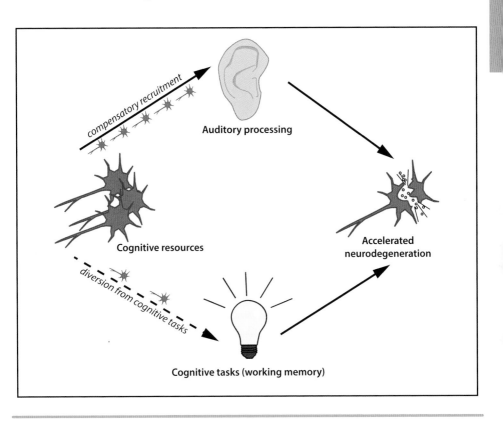

FIGURE 1.30. The Cognitive Load Hypothesis suggests that hearing loss diverts cognitive resources from memory functions to auditory processing. The three hypotheses (Common Cause, Cascade, and Cognitive Load) are not necessarily mutually exclusive; each may play a role in the connection between hearing loss and dementia. Therefore, hypothetically, treating hearing loss (e.g., with cochlear implants or hearing aids) may potentially help prevent, or delay the onset of, dementia (Stahl, 2017).

The Importance of Early Detection

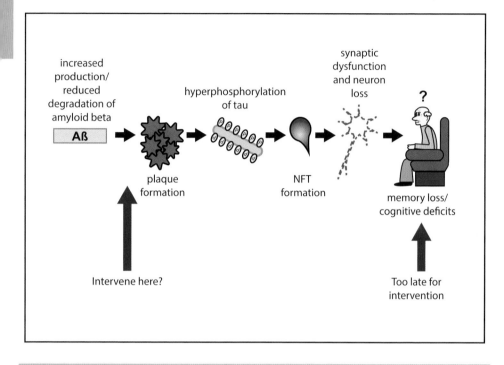

FIGURE 1.31. Until recently, patients could be diagnosed with "possible AD" based solely on clinical assessment and the confirmation of Alzheimer's disease pathology in the brain made only after death. Thus, initiating treatment before the amyloid cascade had progressed beyond the point of irreversibility was an impossibility. However, the last decade has seen tremendous advances in our ability to detect AD pathology in the living patient years before any clinical signs of cognitive impairment or dementia manifest. With these novel techniques, it is now hypothetically possible for potential AD treatments to be tested before the amyloid cascade is irreversible and before AD (or even MCI) is clinically diagnosable. In other words, if the Amyloid Cascade Hypothesis is correct, we now have the ability to possibly prevent, or at least slow, the progression of AD (Cummings, 2011; Fan and Chiu, 2010; Sharma and Singh, 2016).

Magnetic Resonance Imaging

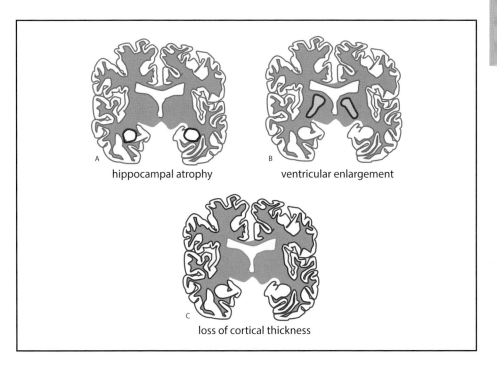

FIGURE 1.32. Magnetic resonance imaging (MRI) can detect atrophy in AD, particularly in the medial temporal lobes (including entorhinal cortex, hippocampus, amygdala, and parahippocampus). Even patients with mild AD may have 20–30% loss in entorhinal cortex volume, 15–25% loss in hippocampal volume, and ventricular enlargement. Thus, by the time a patient begins to exhibit even mild signs of dementia due to AD, damage to the brain may already be extensive and irreversible. Although the brain atrophy seen in AD usually follows a typical pattern, MRI is not diagnostic because atrophy patterns in AD can overlap with those of other diseases and some cases of AD have an atypical presentation (Johnson et al, 2011; Bonifacio and Zamboni, 2016).

FDG-PET

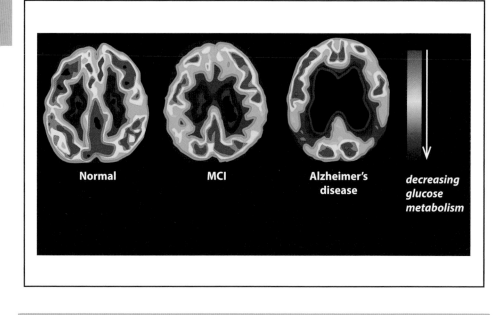

FIGURE 1.33. 18F-2-Fluoro-2-Deoxy-D-Glucose positron emission tomography (FDG-PET) measures glucose metabolism in the brain as an indirect measure of synaptic activity. The FDG-PET abnormalities seen in patients with AD may reflect a number of factors in the brain including mitochondrial dysfunction, oxidative stress, aberrant synaptic plasticity, glial activation and inflammation, reduced cerebral blood flow, and synaptic dysfunction of neuronal death (Johnson et al, 2011).

Amyloid PET

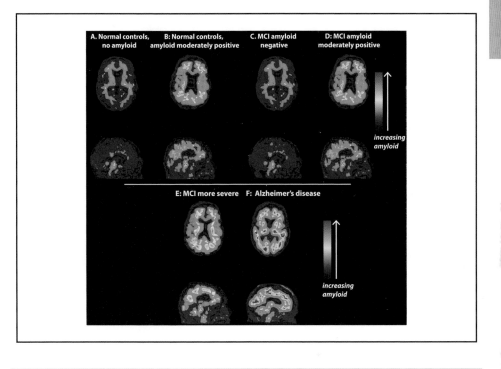

FIGURE 1.34. Several amyloid tracers have been developed; these radioligands bind to Aβ in the brain and can be visualized using positron emission tomography (PET). Although all patients with AD show Aβ pathology while using these amyloid tracers, amyloid PET cannot be used to make a definitive diagnosis of AD because as many as 40% of cognitively normal elderly individuals may have positive amyloid PET results. Cost and availability, as well as disputes regarding what threshold constitutes a "positive" amyloid PET result, have somewhat limited the use of amyloid PET in clinical practice. However, three amyloid tracers (18F-Florbetaben [Neuraceq], 18F-Florbetapir [Amyvid], and 18F-Flutemetamol [Vizamyl]) have been Food and Drug Administration (FDA)-approved to rule out (not diagnose) AD, and several other amyloid tracers are in development. While a positive amyloid PET scan does not necessarily establish a diagnosis of AD, a negative scan indicates that no Aβ pathology is present, thereby demonstrating that AD is not the cause of dementia (Anand and Sabbagh, 2017; Mallik et al, 2017; Villemagne et al, 2017).

Tau PET

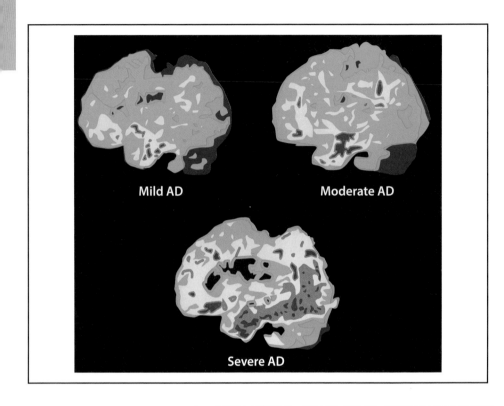

Mild AD

Moderate AD

Severe AD

FIGURE 1.35. Radioligands that bind to tau and can be visualized using PET are also in development. Tau pathology is not unique to AD; thus like amyloid PET, a positive tau PET result is not diagnostic of AD. However, when added to the armamentarium of biomarkers for AD and other dementias, tau PET may greatly aid in the differential diagnosis of dementia (Arendt et al, 2016; Gordon et al, 2016; Villemagne et al, 2017; Kolb and Andres, 2017).

Cerebrospinal Fluid Measures

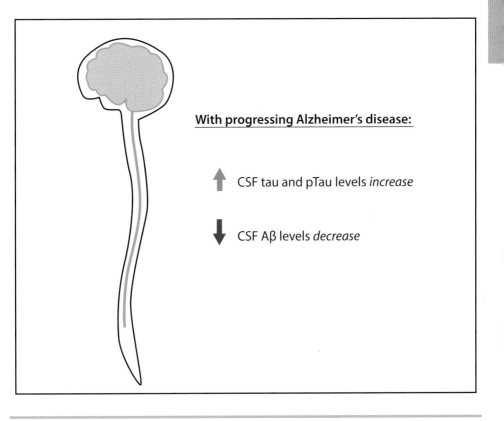

With progressing Alzheimer's disease:

⬆ CSF tau and pTau levels *increase*

⬇ CSF Aβ levels *decrease*

FIGURE 1.36. We now also have the ability to detect AD-related pathology using biomarkers found in the cerebrospinal fluid (CSF). As neurodegeneration in the AD brain increases, so do levels of both tau and phosphorylated tau (pTau) in the CSF. Contrary to this, measures of Aβ are actually decreased in the CSF of patients with AD. This decrease in Aβ is hypothesized to result from increased deposition of Aβ into plaques into the brain and/or decreased production of Aβ as amyloid-producing neurons in the brain die. These CSF measures can also aid in the differential diagnosis of dementia; in patients with positive CSF measures of tau but negative CSF measures of Aβ, the cause of dementia is likely a tauopathy other than Alzheimer's disease (Herukka et al, 2017; Herrmann et al, 2011; Johnson et al, 2011; Simonsen et al, 2017; Spies et al, 2013; Spies et al, 2012).

Progression of AD Pathology, Clinical Symptoms, and Biomarkers

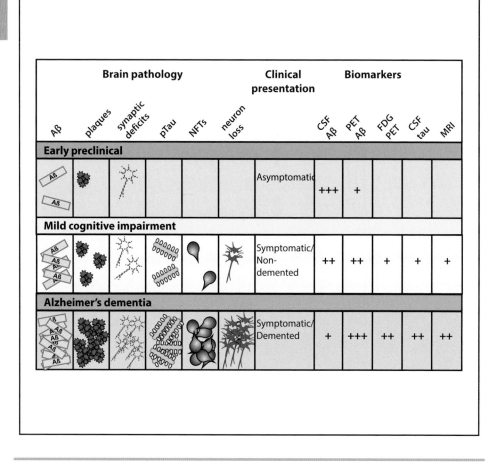

FIGURE 1.37. Alzheimer's pathology may begin decades before the onset of clinical symptoms. As AD pathology progresses, changes in AD biomarkers can also be seen (Albert et al, 2011).

The Retina as a Window to the Brain

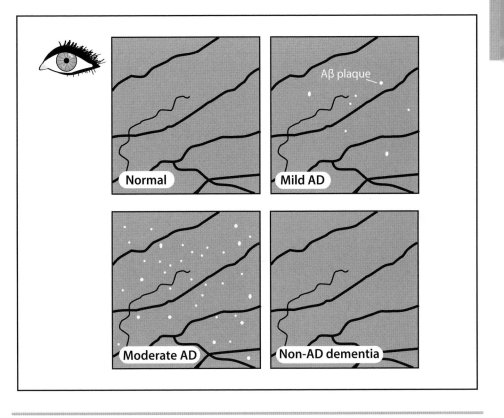

FIGURE 1.38. Given that the retina shares physiological features with the brain, one fascinating technique being developed as a less invasive (compared to CSF, MRI, or PET measures) way to detect AD pathology in the brains of living patients is through retinal imaging. Indeed, it has been shown that curcumin-labeled Aβ plaques can be visualized through retinal scanning and that these retinal plaques correlate well with AD pathology in the brain upon autopsy. Thus, in the near future, this technique may offer a relatively inexpensive method for the early, differential diagnosis of AD that can be easily implemented and performed as part of a routine eye examination (Cheung et al, 2017; Lim et al, 2016; Koronyo et al, 2017).

Sniffing out Alzheimer's Disease

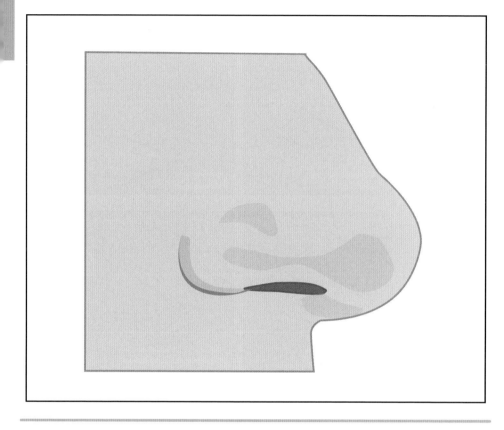

FIGURE 1.39. Deficits in olfaction, especially odor identification, are often robust in patients with mild cognitive impairment (MCI) and may reflect damage to the hippocampus and entorhinal cortex. It has therefore been proposed that olfactory testing may, hypothetically, be used as a non-invasive, fast, inexpensive method to screen for MCI and patients at risk for developing AD (or another dementia where olfactory deficits are also evident, such as dementia with Lewy bodies) (Roalf et al, 2016).

Does the Presence of Aβ Mean Alzheimer's Disease Is Inevitable?

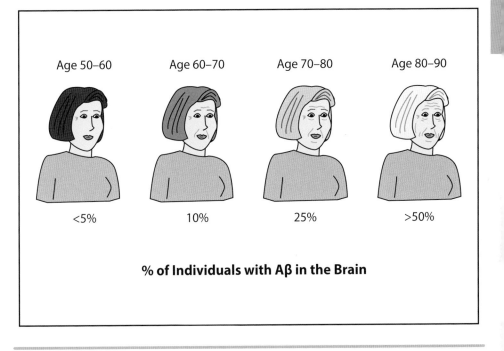

% of Individuals with Aβ in the Brain

(Ages and percentages shown: Age 50–60: <5%; Age 60–70: 10%; Age 70–80: 25%; Age 80–90: >50%)

FIGURE 1.40. Not all individuals with Aβ protein detectable in the brain have Alzheimer's disease. Although the presence of Aβ has been associated with slightly poorer cognitive performance, approximately 25–35% of individuals with Aβ accumulation in the brain perform within normal limits on tests of cognition. Some hypothesize that such individuals may be in the preclinical or prodromal phases of dementia and will inevitably develop dementia should they live long enough (Gurnani and Gavett, 2016; Jack Jr et al, 2017; Mallik et al, 2017; Villemagne et al, 2017).

All-Cause Dementia Diagnosis

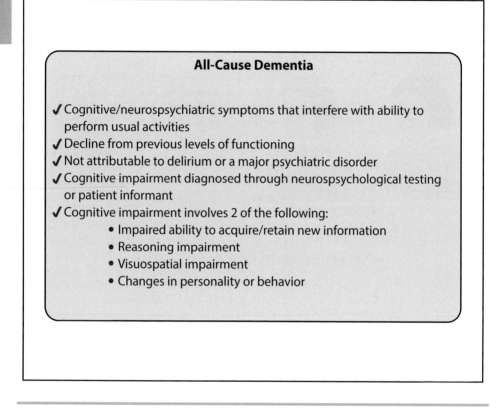

FIGURE 1.41. Dementia can be caused by various pathologies and has differing clinical characteristics; however, all types of dementia share certain clinical features (Grandy, 2012).

Probable Alzheimer's Disease Diagnosis

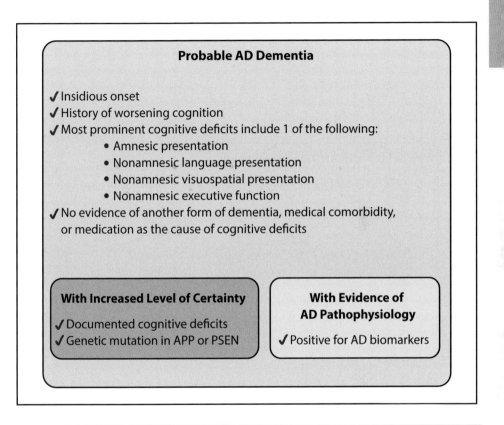

Probable AD Dementia

✓ Insidious onset
✓ History of worsening cognition
✓ Most prominent cognitive deficits include 1 of the following:
  • Amnesic presentation
  • Nonamnesic language presentation
  • Nonamnesic visuospatial presentation
  • Nonamnesic executive function
✓ No evidence of another form of dementia, medical comorbidity, or medication as the cause of cognitive deficits

With Increased Level of Certainty

✓ Documented cognitive deficits
✓ Genetic mutation in APP or PSEN

With Evidence of AD Pathophysiology

✓ Positive for AD biomarkers

FIGURE 1.42. In 2011, the National Institute on Aging and the Alzheimer's Association released new diagnostic guidelines for Alzheimer's disease that incorporate genetics and biomarker evidence of pathology. Although AD can only be officially diagnosed postmortem, these diagnostic guidelines allow for a differential diagnosis to be made with increasing levels of certainty in living patients. Probable AD dementia is diagnosed when the clinical presentation follows a typical course and can be further supported by biomarker and genetic evidence of AD pathology (Grandy, 2012).

Possible Alzheimer's Disease Diagnosis

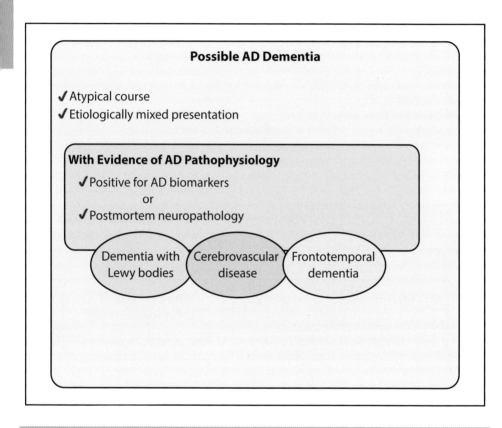

FIGURE 1.43. Often the diagnosis of AD dementia is not clear, typically due to mixed pathological processes contributing to the cognitive dysfunction. In these cases of "mixed dementia," the diagnosis is often possible AD dementia, especially when there is a biomarker or genetic evidence of AD pathology (Grandy, 2012).

Clinical Progression of Alzheimer's Disease

Early/mild: forgetfulness; short-term memory loss; misplaces items; trouble with complicated tasks; searches for words

Middle/moderate: increased language problem; forgets major events; may need help dressing, cooking; may have a decrease in personal hygiene

Late/severe: verbal communication dwindles; needs help eating, bathing; significant long-term memory loss; decline in motor abilities; does not recognize family members

FIGURE 1.44. As AD progresses, behavioral deficits become increasingly severe and the patient's abilities to complete activities of daily living decline. In addition to the memory deficits and cognitive dysfunction, most patients with AD also exhibit other abnormal neuropsychiatric behaviors such as agitation and psychosis. During the later stages of the disease, patients require round-the-clock care. Alzheimer's disease is typically slow in causing actual death; many patients survive a decade or more with severe AD (Alzheimer's Association, 2017).

Mild Cognitive Impairment

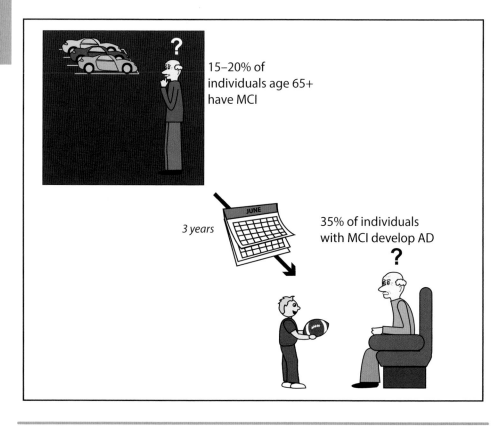

15–20% of individuals age 65+ have MCI

3 years

35% of individuals with MCI develop AD

FIGURE 1.45. Mild cognitive impairment (MCI) denotes the presence of mild cognitive decline that does not significantly affect the ability to carry out activities of daily living and does not meet the threshold for dementia. Although MCI is evident in the early, prodromal stages of AD, not all patients with MCI will go on to develop AD and, in fact, many individuals with MCI can return to healthy cognition with proper treatment. For example, patients with a major depressive disorder often present with MCI but, with proper antidepressant treatment, symptoms of MCI often improve or remit. One of the great efforts on the part of Alzheimer's researchers is determining what factors (e.g., positive AD biomarker evidence) might help to predict which patients will progress from MCI to AD (Alzheimer's Association, 2017; Alexopoulos et al, 2016; Allan et al, 2017; Burmester et al, 2016; Herukka et al, 2017; Mallik et al, 2017; Pascoal et al, 2017; Pandya et al, 2016).

Differential Diagnosis: Clinical Presentation

Normal Aging	AD (Alzheimer's disease)	VaD (Vascular dementia)	DLB (Dementia w/ Lewy bodies)	FTLD (Frontotemporal lobe degeneration)
• Reduced speed of mental processing and choice reaction times • Benign forgetfulness that is mild, inconsistent, and not associated with functional impairment	• Short-term memory loss • Impaired executive function • Difficulty with activities of daily living • Time and spatial disorientation • Language impairment, personality changes	• Impaired abstraction, mental flexibility, processing speed, and working memory • Verbal memory is better preserved • Slower cognitive decline • Dementia occurs within several months of a stroke	• Visual hallucinations • Spontaneous parkinsonism • Cognitive fluctuations • Visuospatial, attention, and executive function deficits are worse • Memory impairment is not as severe • Earlier presentation of psychosis and personality changes • Rapid eye movement (REM) sleep disturbances	• Progressive behavioral and personality changes that impair social conduct (apathy, disinhibition, etc.) • Language impairment • Possibly preserved episodic memory

FIGURE 1.46. The most common causes of dementia, including Alzheimer's disease (AD), vascular dementia (VaD), dementia with Lewy bodies (DLB), and frontotemporal lobar degeneration (FTLD), typically present with clinical symptoms that differ from one another and from the mild cognitive decline often seen in healthy aging. Each of these common forms of dementia is discussed in more detail in subsequent chapters (Tarawneh and Holtzman, 2012; Weintraub et al, 2012; Ritter et al, 2017).

Differential Diagnosis: Neuroimaging

	AD	VaD	DLB	FTLD
MRI	Medial temporal lobe atrophy	Medial temporal lobe atrophy; white matter abnormalities	Medial temporal lobe atrophy	Medial temporal lobe atrophy
FDG-PET	Temporoparietal cortices	Fronto-subcortical networks	Parieto-occipital and temporoparietal cortices	Frontotemporal cortices

FIGURE 1.47. The most common causes of dementia, including Alzheimer's disease (AD), vascular dementia (VaD), dementia with Lewy bodies (DLB), and frontotemporal lobar degeneration (FTLD), also each have distinct features visible through magnetic resonance imaging (MRI) and fluorodeoxyglucose—positron emission tomography (FDG-PET) (Johnson et al, 2011).

Clinical Assessment of Dementia

Short Blessed Test (SBT)	6-item weighted version of the Information–Memory–Concentration Test; usually completed in 5 min; good correlation with AD pathology
Mini-Mental Status Examination (MMSE)	19 items measuring orientation, memory, concentration, language, and praxis; most widely used screening test
Alzheimer's Disease Assessment Scale—cognitive subscale (ADAS-cog)	A 20-minute, 70-point scale with 11–14 items that tests memory, language, orientation, and praxis
7-Minute Screen	4 tests (orientation, memory, clock drawing, and verbal fluency)
General Practitioner Assessment of Cognition (GPCOG)	A 6-item screening test similar to the SBT, a clock drawing, and a 5-item informant questionnaire
Montreal Cognitive Assessment (MoCA)	An 8-item, 20-minute evaluation measuring attention, concentration, executive function, language, conceptual thinking, and orientation; 30 points total with 26 or above considered normal
Clinical Dementia Rating (CDR Scale)	A 5-point scale characterizing 6 domains of cognitive and functional performance including memory, orientation, judgment and problem solving, community affairs, home and hobbies, and personal care

FIGURE 1.48. Neuropsychological assessment, including cognitive measures of memory, executive functioning, and activities of daily living, should be done in all patients with suspected dementia in order to aid diagnosis and track disease progression. As such, there is a variety of brief cognitive screening tests available for assessing dementia (Yang et al, 2016; Tarawneh and Holtzman, 2012).

Currently Available Treatments for Alzheimer's Disease

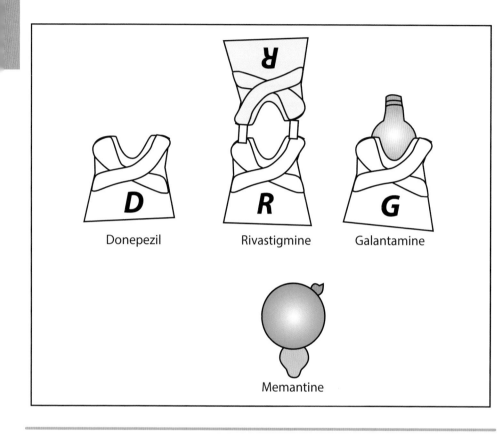

Donepezil

Rivastigmine

Galantamine

Memantine

FIGURE 1.49. Available treatments, including the cholinesterase inhibitors donepezil, rivastigmine, galantamine, and the *N*-methyl-D-aspartate (NMDA) receptor antagonist memantine, may slow progression of AD for a short period of time; however, these existing treatments are ultimately unable to halt progression of the neuronal destruction, memory loss, cognitive deficits, and other neuropsychiatric symptoms of AD (including agitation and psychosis). Although these available treatments provide only moderate symptom relief rather than modifying the clinical course of AD, they can delay institutionalization for up to 2 years. A tremendous effort is underway to find an effective treatment for AD (Stahl, 2013; Geldmacher et al, 2003).

Cholinergic Neurotransmission

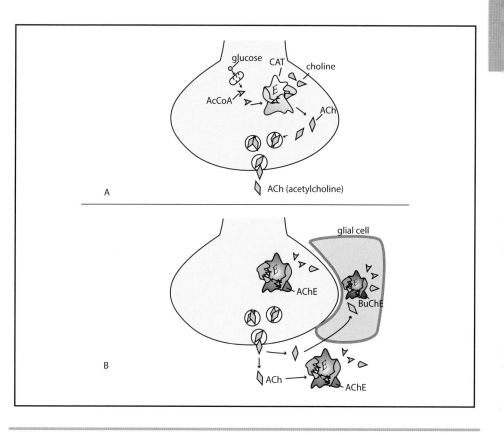

FIGURE 1.50. (A) Acetylcholine (ACh) is formed when two precursors—choline and acetyl coenzyme A (AcCoA)—interact with the synthetic enzyme choline acetyltransferase (CAT). Choline is derived from dietary and intraneuronal sources, and AcCoA is made from glucose in the mitochondria of the neuron. (B) Acetylcholine's action can be terminated by two different enzymes: acetylcholinesterase (AChE), which is present both intracellularly and extracellularly, and butyrylcholinesterase (BuChE), which is particularly present in glial cells. Both enzymes convert acetylcholine into choline, which is then transported out of the synaptic cleft and back into the presynaptic neuron via the choline transporter. Once inside the presynaptic neuron, choline can be recycled into acetylcholine and then packaged into vesicles by the vesicular transporter for acetylcholine (VAChT) (Stahl, 2013).

Donepezil

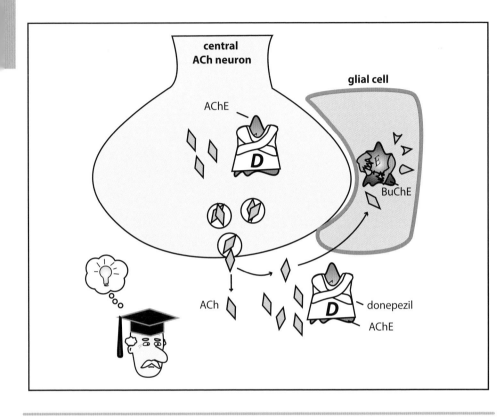

FIGURE 1.51. Donepezil is a reversible, long-acting selective inhibitor of acetylcholinesterase (AChE). It is FDA-approved for the treatment of mild to severe AD and is available as a once-daily formulation. The most notable side effects associated with donepezil are transient gastrointestinal issues. Donepezil inhibits the enzyme AChE, which is present both in the central nervous system (CNS) and peripherally. Central cholinergic neurons are important for the regulation of memory; thus, in the CNS, the boost of acetylcholine caused by AChE blockade contributes to improved cognitive functioning. Peripheral cholinergic neurons in the gut are involved in gastrointestinal effects; thus, the boost in peripheral acetylcholine caused by AChE blockade may contribute to gastrointestinal side effects (Stahl, 2013).

BuChE: butyrylcholinesterase

Rivastigmine

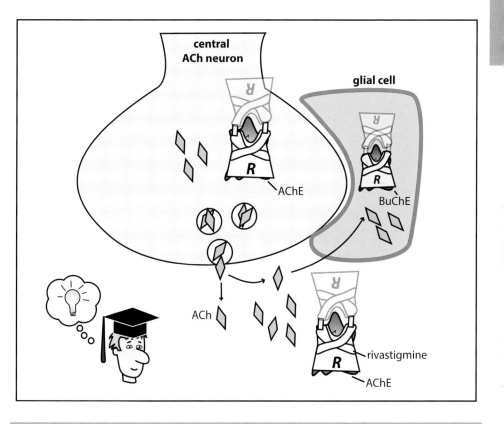

FIGURE 1.52. Rivastigmine is a pseudo-irreversible, intermediate-acting inhibitor of neuronal acetylcholinesterase (AChE) and glial butyrylcholinesterase (BuChE) that is FDA-approved for the treatment of mild-to-moderate AD. In particular, rivastigmine appears to be somewhat selective for AChE in the cortex and hippocampus—two regions important for memory—over other areas of the brain. Rivastigmine's blockade of BuChE in glia may also contribute to enhanced acetylcholine levels. Inhibition of BuChE may be more important in later stages of disease because as more cholinergic neurons die and gliosis occurs, BuChE activity increases. Side effects, most commonly gastrointestinal in nature, can be reduced with the transdermal formulation (Stahl, 2013).

Galantamine

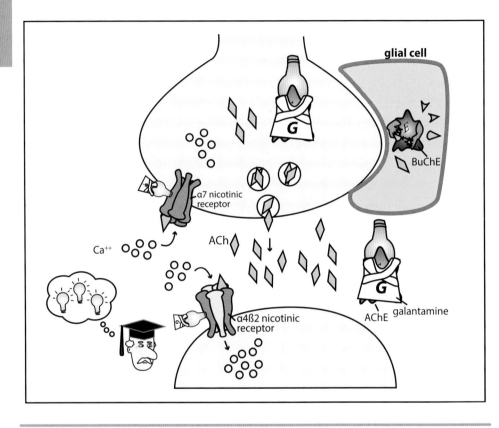

FIGURE 1.53. Galantamine is another acetylcholinesterase inhibitor; however, it is unique among cholinesterase inhibitors in that it is also a positive allosteric modulator (PAM) at nicotinic cholinergic receptors, which means it can boost the effects of acetylcholine at these receptors. Thus galantamine's second action as a PAM at nicotinic receptors could theoretically enhance its primary action as a cholinesterase inhibitor. Galantamine is FDA-approved for the treatment of mild-to-moderate AD and is available in a once-daily formulation (Stahl, 2013).

Cholinesterase Inhibitors in Practice

Drug	Doses Per Day	BuChE Inhibition	Nausea	Vomiting	Diarrhea	Anorexia
Donepezil	1	-	+	+	+	+
Rivastigmine	2	+	++++	+++	+	++
Galantamine	1 or 2	-	++	++	+	+

FIGURE 1.54. Donepezil is generally used first. Surprisingly, if not effective, another cholinesterase inhibitor (e.g., rivastigmine; galantamine) can benefit the patient in 50% of cases. Thus, therapeutic failure is not a class effect with these drugs (Stahl, 2013; Ohta et al, 2017).

Glutamatergic Neurotransmission in AD: Part 1

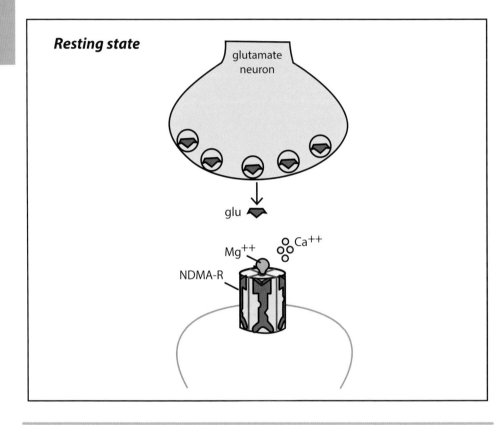

FIGURE 1.55. In the resting state, glutamate is quiet and *N*-methyl-D-aspartate (NMDA) receptors (NMDA-Rs) are blocked by magnesium (Stahl, 2013).

Glutamatergic Neurotransmission in AD: Part 2

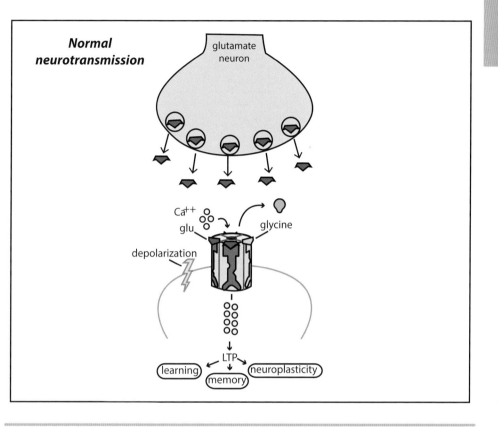

FIGURE 1.56. With normal neurotransmission, glutamate binds to NMDA receptors and, if the postsynaptic receptor is depolarized and glycine is simultaneously bound to the NMDA receptors, the channel opens and allows ion influx (Stahl, 2013).

LTP: long-term potentiation

Glutamatergic Neurotransmission in AD: Part 3

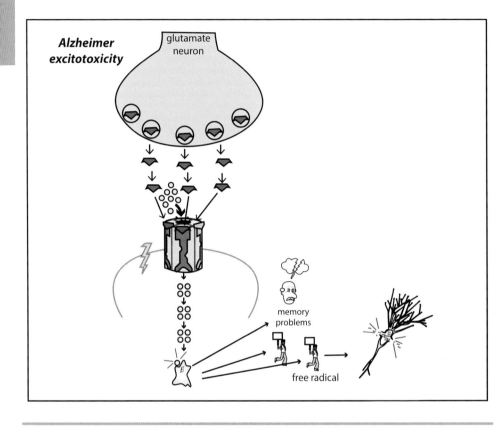

FIGURE 1.57. If amyloid's synaptic effects include downregulating the glutamate transporter, inhibiting glutamate reuptake, or enhancing glutamate release, this could cause a steady leak of glutamate and result in excessive calcium influx in postsynaptic neurons, which in the short term may cause memory problems and in the long term may cause accumulation of free radicals and thus destruction of neurons (Stahl, 2013).

Glutamatergic Neurotransmission in AD: Part 4

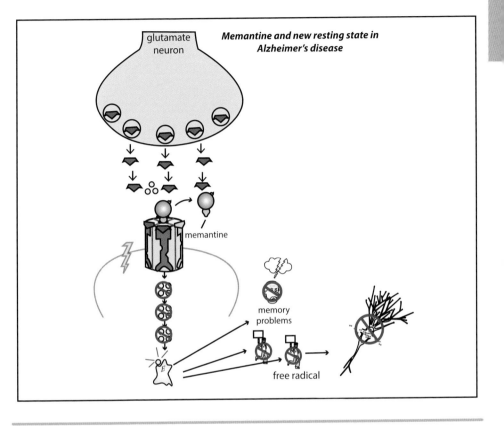

FIGURE 1.58. Memantine is a non-competitive low-affinity *N*-methyl-ᴅ-aspartate (NMDA) receptor antagonist that binds to the magnesium site when the channel is open. Memantine blocks the downstream effects of tonic glutamate release by "plugging" the NMDA ion channel and thus may improve memory and prevent neurodegeneration (Stahl, 2013).

Glutamatergic Neurotransmission in AD: Part 5

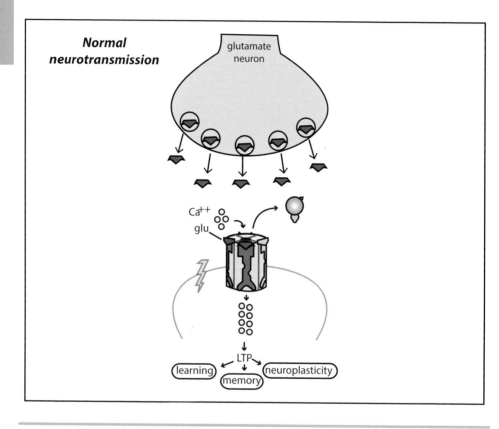

FIGURE 1.59. Memantine has low affinity for NMDA receptors; therefore, when there is a phasic burst of glutamate and depolarization occurs, this is enough to remove memantine from the ion channel and thus allow normal neurotransmission (Stahl, 2013).

Treatment Algorithm for Alzheimer's Disease

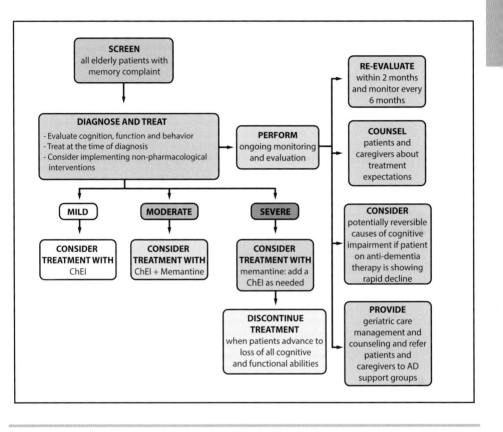

FIGURE 1.60. In addition to pharmacological treatments for Alzheimer's disease, non-pharmacological interventions such as cognitive training, reality orientation, and cognitive stimulation therapy may improve cognitive functioning and quality of life in some patients with AD (Sadowsky and Galvin, 2012; Ballard et al, 2011; Gehres et al, 2016).

ChEI: cholinesterase inhibitor

Novel Potential Treatments for Alzheimer's Disease

Agents Targeting Aβ Pathology

Anti-amyloid antibodies
Active Aβ immunization
β-secretase inhibitors
Y-secretase inhibitors
α-secretase promotors
Aβ aggregation inhibitors

Agents Targeting Metabolic Factors

Intranasal insulin
Statins
Anti-diabetes drugs
Probiotics

Agents Modulating Neurotransmission

Serotonin 5HT6 antagonists
Histamine H3 antagonists
5HT2A antagonists

Agents Targeting Tau Pathology

Anti-tau antibodies
Active tau immunization
Tau aggregation inhibitors
Microtubule stabilizers
Tau phosphorylation inhibitors

Agents Targeting Inflammation

COX-2 selective compounds
Curcumin
Docosahexanoic acid
Resveratrol
Omega-3 and omega-6 fatty acids
Vitamin E

Others

RAGE inhibitors
Calcium channel blockers
Estrogen

FIGURE 1.61. There are numerous agents currently being studied as potential disease-modifying medications for AD. Primarily, these agents fall into five main categories targeting different aspects of Alzheimer's pathology: amyloid pathology; tau pathology; inflammation; metabolic factors; and neurotransmitter modulation. Some of these novel agents (notably the anti-amyloid antibodies and secretase inhibitors) have made it as far as Phase III clinical testing; however, most of these later-stage trials have failed to show efficacy or have caused side effects serious enough to halt testing. There is a strong consensus that in order for an agent to actually modify Alzheimer's disease course, it will need to be initiated at the very earliest stages of pathology—likely before a patient actually shows any clinical signs of dementia. In this regard, the most recent clinical trials, which employ amyloid and tau biomarkers to detect Alzheimer's disease pathology, may demonstrate more promising results (Arbor et al, 2016; Bronzuoli et al, 2016; Ferrero et al, 2017; MacLeod et al, 2015; Mendiola-Precoma et al, 2016; Panza et al, 2016; Ruthirakuhan et al, 2016; Yan, 2016).

Passive Immunization with Anti-Amyloid Antibodies

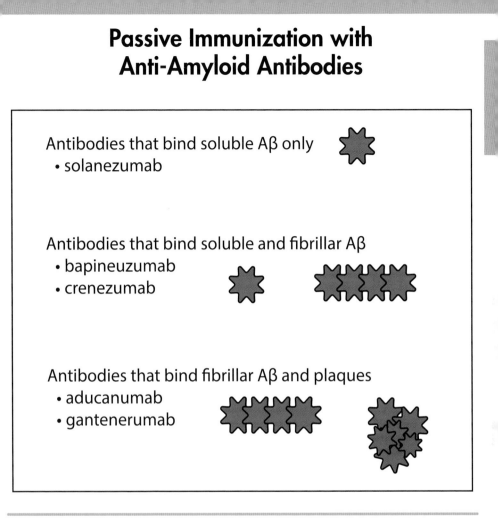

FIGURE 1.62. Antibody-based immunotherapies consist of monoclonal antibodies developed to bind amyloid beta (Aβ) proteins. However, the various anti-amyloid immunotherapies currently in clinical testing are binding to different portions or conformations of the amyloid beta peptide and are thought to remove Aβ from the brain via three hypothesized mechanisms. These mechanisms are peripheral sink; disaggregation; and microglia engagement and phagocytosis. Unfortunately, one issue that has been seen in trials using anti-Aβ antibodies has been the appearance of amyloid-related imaging abnormalities (ARIA) using MRI. These ARIA are thought to represent edema or microhemorrhages caused by the removal of Aβ from blood vessel walls and subsequent leakage of water or blood into the brain (Godyn et al, 2016; Panza et al, 2016; Mallik et al, 2017).

Anti-Amyloid Antibodies: Phagocytosis

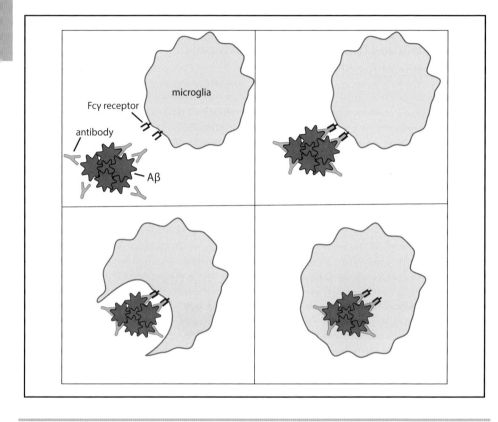

FIGURE 1.63. During microglia engagement and phagocytosis, one portion of the antibody binds to the amyloid beta peptide whereas the Fc portion of the antibody serves as a beacon to call in microglia, the phagocytic cells of the central nervous system. After an antibody binds to amyloid beta protein, Fc-gamma receptors found on microglia bind to the Fc portion of the antibodies. The binding of Fc-gamma receptors to the Fc portion of the antibody causes microglia to engulf amyloid plaques, resulting in the removal of amyloid beta from the brain (Godyn et al, 2016; Panza et al, 2016).

Anti-Amyloid Antibodies: Peripheral Sink

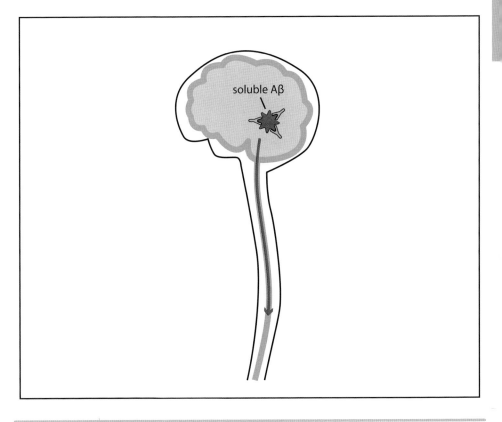

FIGURE 1.64. According to the peripheral sink mechanism, anti-amyloid antibodies bind to the soluble amyloid beta protein before it can aggregate into plaques and cause the removal of that amyloid beta from the brain to the CSF. Consequently, this clearance of soluble, unaggregated amyloid beta hypothetically prevents the growth of amyloid beta plaques (Godyn et al, 2016; Panza et al, 2016).

Anti-Amyloid Antibodies: Disaggregation

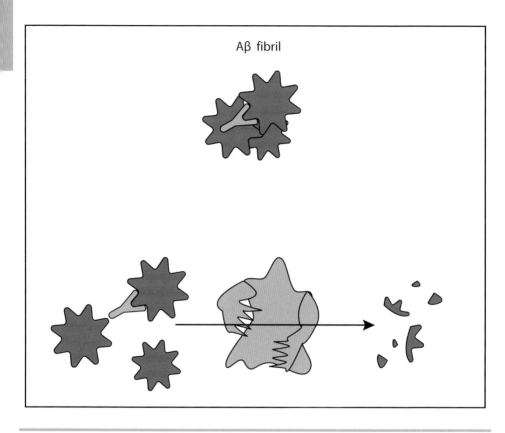

Aβ fibril

FIGURE 1.65. With the disaggregation mechanism, binding of antibodies to insoluble amyloid beta fibrils causes a disruption of the tertiary structure of the amyloid beta protein. This disruption may hypothetically allow amyloid beta degrading enzymes to access and break down amyloid beta proteins (Godyn et al, 2016; Panza et al, 2016).

Active Aβ Immunization

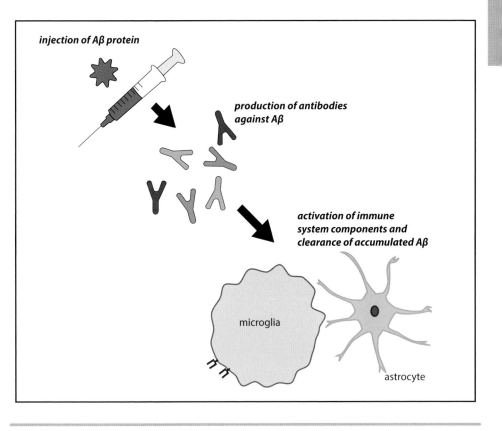

FIGURE 1.66. Active vaccination is another type of immunization that is being investigated for AD. With active immunization, the Aβ protein (either full length or a fragment thereof) is injected, typically with an adjuvant designed to spark the natural immune system. Earliest trials with such vaccines had to be halted due to the induction of severe inflammatory reactions including encephalitis, and many hypothesize that these inflammatory reactions were stimulated by using adjuvants that activated a T-helper cell 1 (Th1) cell response. Th1 immune responses involve more proinflammatory molecules (e.g., cytokines) whereas Th2 cell responses tend to be anti-inflammatory. Researchers are now pursuing Aβ vaccination using Th2-stimulating adjuvants (Wisniewski and Drummond, 2016; Marciani, 2015).

Alpha-Secretase Promotors

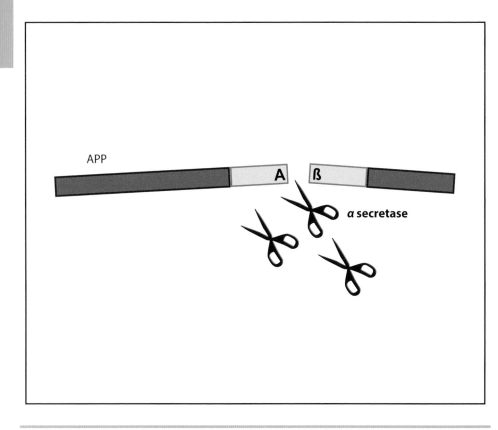

FIGURE 1.67. One potential mechanism for reducing the production of Aβ involves promoting α-secretase cleavage of the amyloid precursor protein (APP). As previously discussed, α-secretase cuts APP within the sequence containing Aβ (i.e., the non-amyloidogenic pathway), thereby precluding the formation of the Aβ peptide. Several agents, including the Monoamine oxidase inhibitor (MAOI) selegiline, the statin atorvastatin, the gamma-aminobutyric acid (GABA) modulator etazolate, the serotonin 5HT4 agonist PRX-03140, the green tea polyphenolic compound epigallocatechin-gallate, the protein kinase modulator bryostatin, and melatonin have been shown to increase α-secretase activity (MacLeod et al, 2015; Mendiola-Precoma et al, 2016).

Beta-Secretase Inhibitors

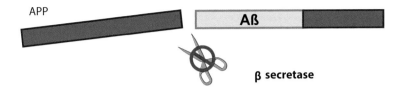

BACE Inhibitor	Clinical Trial Phase
Verubecestat	III
AZD3293	III
E2609	III
CNP520	II / III
JNJ-548611	II / III
CTS21166	I
HPP854	I

FIGURE 1.68. The idea behind using agents that block β-secretase (a.k.a. β-amyloid cleaving enzyme or BACE) is that prevention of cleavage of the amyloid precursor protein (APP) by BACE will inhibit the amyloidogenic APP processing pathway and stop the formation of Aβ protein. Unfortunately, many trials of BACE inhibitors have been halted due to safety concerns, including liver toxicity. The adverse effects of BACE inhibition likely have to do with some of the other processes that BACE is involved in, including muscle spindle formation, myelination, sodium homeostasis, neuronal migration, neurogenesis, and astrogenesis (MacLeod et al, 2015; Ruthirakuhan et al, 2016; Yan, 2016).

Gamma-Secretase Inhibitors

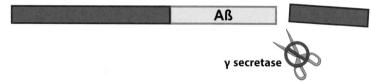

γ-Secretase Inhibitor	Clinical Trial Phase
Semagacestat	III
Avagacestat	II
EVP0962	II
NIC515	II
γ-Secretase Modulator	**Clinical Trial Phase**
Tarenflurbil	III
CHF5074	II
NIC515	II

FIGURE 1.69. As with BACE inhibition, the idea behind inhibiting γ-secretase is to reduce amyloidogenic processing of APP. Unfortunately, as with many of the BACE inhibitors, most of the studies of γ-secretase inhibitors have been terminated due to safety concerns including skin cancer and the worsening of cognition. In addition to APP, γ-secretase has many other substrates, most notably Notch (a protein important for neurogenesis). Researchers are now working on Notch-sparing γ-secretase inhibitors as well as γ-secretase modulators that may shift γ-secretase processing of APP so that smaller (e.g., Aβ40) rather than larger more toxic (e.g., Aβ42) isoforms are produced (Arbor et al, 2016; MacLeod et al, 2015; Mendiola-Precoma et al, 2016; Ruthirakuhan et al, 2016).

Targeting Tau Pathology

Tau Vaccination
AADvac1
ACI-35
RG7345
Tau Aggregation Inhibition
Leucomethylthioninium
Methylthioninium chloride
Microtubule Stabilization
TPI-287
Davunetide
Epothilone

FIGURE 1.70. In addition to novel therapies that target production, degradation, or aggregation of Aβ, exploration of many of these strategies is also being directed towards tau protein. Trials with these agents are still primarily in the early phases; however, if successful, such tau-modifying treatments would potentially be applicable in other tauopathies, such as frontotemporal lobar degeneration (Mendiola-Precoma et al, 2016; Panza et al, 2016; Ruthirakuhan et al, 2016).

Estrogen

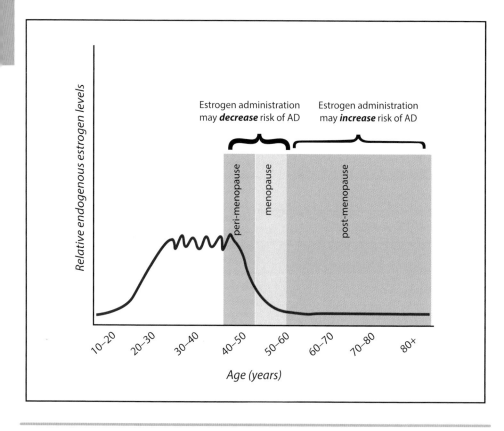

FIGURE 1.71. There are some data, albeit somewhat conflicting, that suggest that estrogen administration in peri- or post-menopausal women may lower the risk of developing AD. However, it appears that the timing of estrogen initiation, as well as apolipoprotein E (APOE) genotype, may be crucial. If delivered during the peri-menopausal phase or shortly after the onset of menopause, estrogen seems protective; however, when administered well after menopause is complete, estrogen seems to actually increase one's risk of developing AD. In terms of APOE genotype, estrogen administration may hypothetically convey the most protection to women who have APOE2 or APOE3 rather than those with APOE4 (Depypere et al, 2016).

5HT6 Receptors

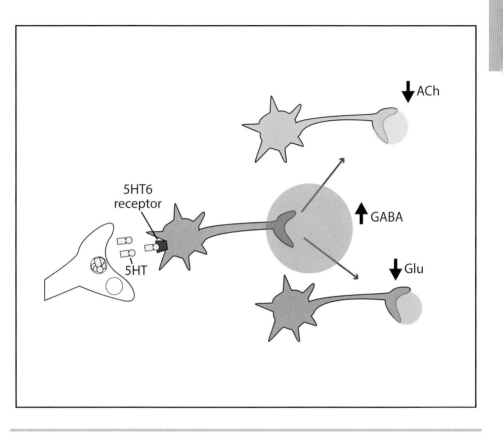

FIGURE 1.72. The serotonin 5HT6 receptor is abundantly located in brain regions associated with memory, including the hippocampus, frontal and entorhinal cortices, nucleus accumbens, and striatum. Binding of serotonin (5HT) to 5HT6 receptors on GABAergic neurons leads to release of GABA on cholinergic (ACh) and glutamatergic (Glu) neurons, causing the inhibition of ACh and Glu release (Ferrero et al, 2017; Atri et al, 2018).

5HT6 Antagonists

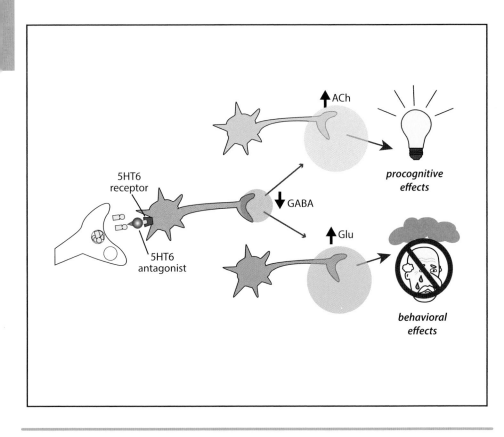

FIGURE 1.73. Antagonism of 5HT6 receptors is hypothesized to lead to disinhibition of both cholinergic (ACh) and glutamatergic (Glu) neurons, thereby improving memory (as well as depression and anxiety—two other frequently exhibited symptoms in dementia). Indeed, agents that modulate the 5HT6 receptor are actively being explored, with some preliminary data suggesting efficacy in improving memory although disappointing results have more recently emerged (Ferrero et al, 2017; Atri et al, 2018).

Lewy Body Dementias and Other Synucleinopathies

Although Alzheimer's disease is the most common cause of dementia, dementia with Lewy bodies (DLB) is another common cause of dementia. In fact, DLB and Parkinson's disease dementia (PDD) account for 10–15% of all cases of dementia. However, only an estimated 20% of patients have "pure" DLB; approximately 80% of patients will also have pathological features of other dementias, namely Alzheimer's disease pathology (Thomas et al, 2017; Yang and Yu, 2017; Karantzoulis and Galvin, 2011). In this chapter, we will discuss the neurobiology and diagnosis of DLB and PDD (collectively known as Lewy body dementias [LBDs]) and other synucleinopathies as well as the hypothesized relationship between Alzheimer's and Parkinson's. For strategies to ameliorate some of the secondary behavioral symptoms often associated with synucleinopathies and other dementias, the reader is directed to Chapter 5.

Alpha-Synuclein

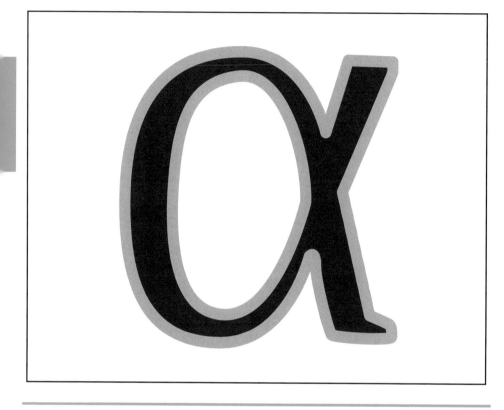

FIGURE 2.1. Alpha-synuclein (αSyn) is the pathologic protein that aggregates in Lewy body dementias (LBDs), including dementia with Lewy bodies (DLB) and Parkinson's disease dementia (PDD), as well as multiple system atrophy (MSA). Although LBD, PDD, and MSA may all present with chronic, progressive decline in motor, cognitive, behavioral, and autonomic functions, the clinical manifestations of these different "synucleinopathies" vary depending on the primary location and subsequent progression of αSyn aggregation. (Dugger and Dickson, 2017; Yang and Yu, 2017; Azizi and Azizi, 2017; Benskey et al, 2016).

Alpha-Synuclein: Normal Function

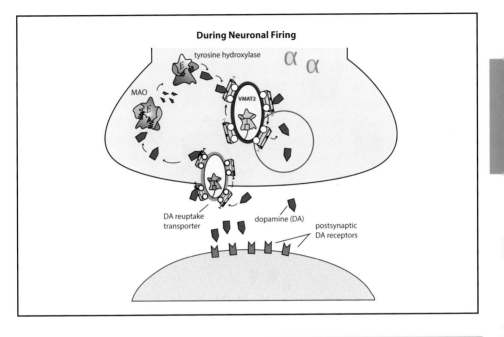

FIGURE 2.2. The exact physiological function(s) of αSyn has yet to be realized; however, αSyn is a ubiquitous protein found throughout the central and peripheral nervous systems; it has been hypothesized that αSyn plays an integral role in the maintenance of synaptic neurotransmission, particularly that of dopaminergic neurotransmission. During neuronal firing, αSyn is dispersed from the presynaptic terminal, leaving tyrosine hydroxylase (the enzyme involved in dopamine [DA] biosynthesis) disinhibited and thus increasing de novo DA synthesis (Dugger and Dickson, 2017; Yang and Yu, 2017; Azizi and Azizi, 2017; Benskey et al, 2016).

MAO: Monoamine oxidase; VMAT: vesicular monoamine transporter

Alpha-Synuclein: Normal Function

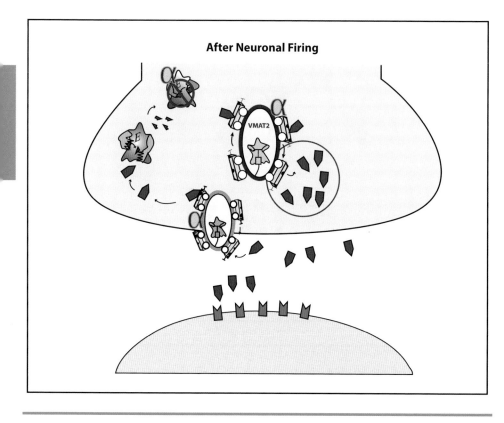

FIGURE 2.3. After completion of neuronal firing, αSyn is replenished in the presynaptic terminal where it inhibits tyrosine hydroxylase (decreasing DA synthesis), increases packaging of DA into vesicles via the vesicular monoamine transporter (VMAT), and modulates the activity of the dopamine transporter (DAT), thereby altering DA levels within the synapse. Together these actions, along with the involvement of αSyn being a factor in the formation and regulation of synaptic vesicles, suggest that αSyn plays an important role in maintaining presynaptic DA levels both during and between neuronal stimulation (Dugger and Dickson, 2017; Yang and Yu, 2017; Azizi and Azizi, 2017; Benskey et al, 2016).

Pathological Alpha-Synuclein

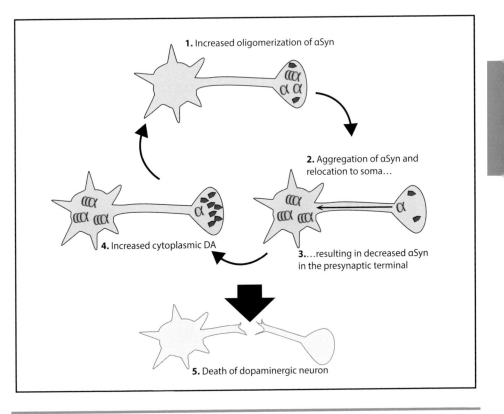

FIGURE 2.4. Each of the synucleinopathies (dementia with Lewy bodies, Parkinson's disease dementia, and multiple system atrophy) is pathologically characterized by (1) oligomerization and (2) aggregation of αSyn. Although it is not entirely clear what initially causes this oligomerization and aggregation of αSyn, several factors including genetics, inflammatory particles, other pathological proteins (e.g., tau or Aβ), and high levels of dopamine (DA) can induce oligomerization of αSyn within axon terminals and lead to its redistribution from the presynaptic terminal to the soma. In a vicious cycle, (3) as αSyn aggregates and is no longer sufficiently present in the presynaptic terminal (where it is needed to regulate dopaminergic neurotransmission), (4) cytoplasmic DA levels increase, leading to further αSyn oligomerization. Not only may these αSyn oligomers directly trigger cell death, elevated cytoplasmic levels of DA are also neurotoxic; ultimately, (5) the result is the death of dopaminergic neurons (Benskey et al, 2016).

Lewy Bodies and Lewy Neurites

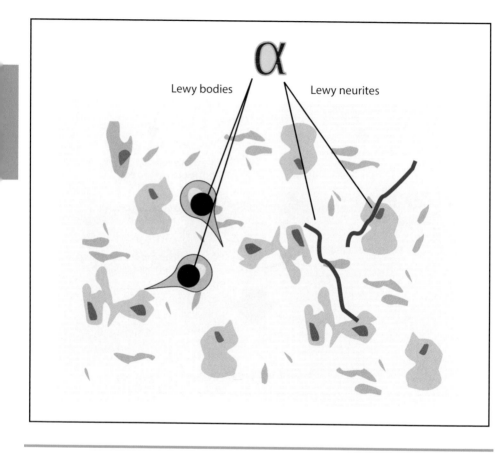

FIGURE 2.5. As discussed, pathological αSyn aggregates and is redistributed from the presynaptic terminal to the soma, especially in dopaminergic neurons. In both dementia with Lewy bodies (DLB) and Parkinson's disease dementia (PDD), these aggregates form Lewy bodies and Lewy neurites that are observable upon histopathological staining. In addition to αSyn, Lewy bodies and Lewy neurites may also contain various other proteins such as neurofilaments, parkin, and ubiquitin (Alafuzoff and Hartikainen, 2017; Azizi and Azizi, 2017; Dugger and Dickson, 2017).

Alpha-Synuclein in the Periphery

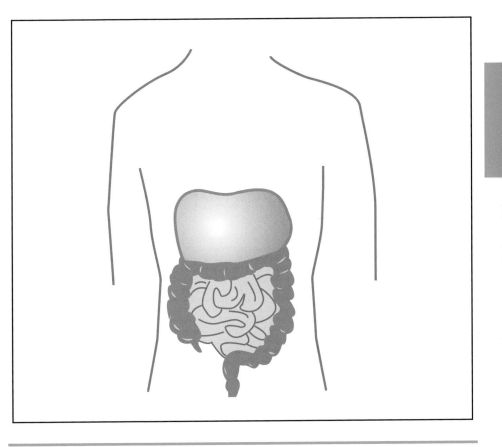

FIGURE 2.6. Not only does αSyn accumulate as Lewy bodies with the nigrostriatal in Parkinson's disease (PD, accounting for the motor symptoms), pathological αSyn also aggregates outside of the central nervous system (CNS), including the enteric nervous system—often years before CNS pathology becomes apparent. It is hypothesized that this αSyn accumulation within the enteric nervous system is the pathological substrate for the gastrointestinal issues commonly experienced in patients with Lewy body disorders, often years before the onset of clinically identifiable motor symptoms (Benskey et al, 2016).

Parkinson's Disease

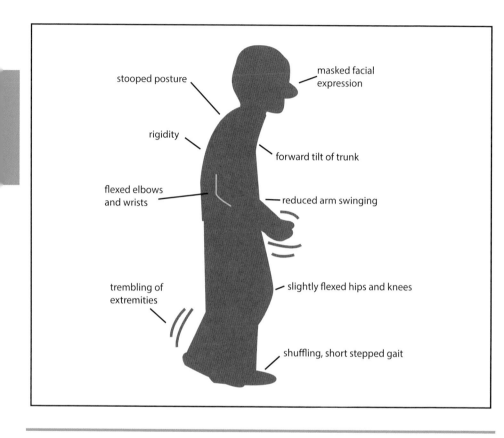

FIGURE 2.7. Worldwide, Parkinson's disease (PD) affects ~2% of individuals age 70 years and older, with a mean age-of-onset of 65 years (although onset has been reported as young as 38 years of age and as old as 87 years of age). Although the characteristic clinical feature of PD is motor dysfunction (such as bradykinesia, rigidity, postural instability, and tremor) due to loss of nigrostriatal dopaminergic neurons, most patients with PD also exhibit a myriad of non-motor symptoms, including olfactory impairments, sleep disturbances, gastrointestinal issues, depression, psychosis, cognitive impairment, and dementia (due to pathological processes outside of the nigrostriatal area). In fact, non-motor symptoms are often the first symptoms to manifest, in many cases long before the onset of motor dysfunction (Alafuzoff and Hartikainen, 2017; Delgado-Morales and Esteller, 2017; Jellinger et al, 2018; Xu et al, 2016; Yang and Yu, 2017).

Parkinson's Disease Diagnosis

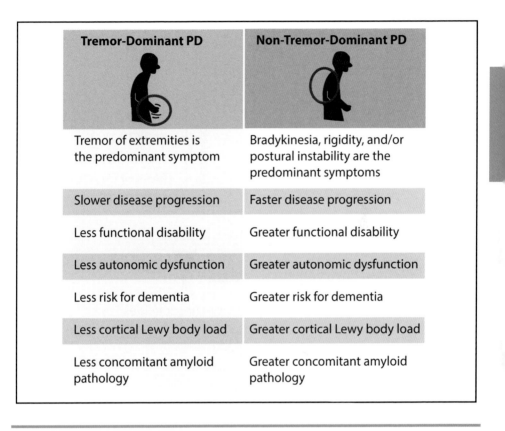

Tremor-Dominant PD	Non-Tremor-Dominant PD
Tremor of extremities is the predominant symptom	Bradykinesia, rigidity, and/or postural instability are the predominant symptoms
Slower disease progression	Faster disease progression
Less functional disability	Greater functional disability
Less autonomic dysfunction	Greater autonomic dysfunction
Less risk for dementia	Greater risk for dementia
Less cortical Lewy body load	Greater cortical Lewy body load
Less concomitant amyloid pathology	Greater concomitant amyloid pathology

FIGURE 2.8. Based on the clinical presentation of motor symptoms, PD is classified as either tremor-dominant PD or non-tremor-dominant (akinetic/rigid) PD, although some patients may present with mixture phenotype. Tremor-dominant PD typically has a slower rate of progression and less functional disability compared to the non-tremor subtype (Alafuzoff and Hartikainen, 2017; Jellinger et al, 2018).

Parkinson's Disease Risk

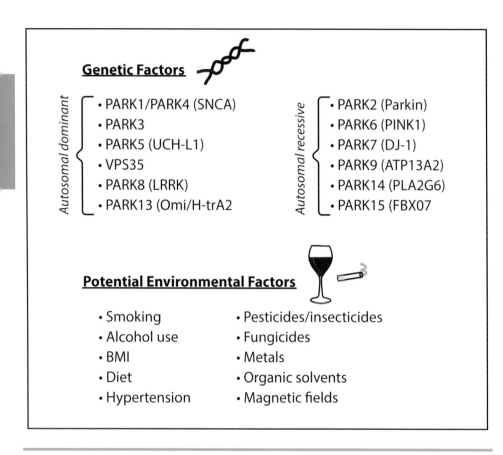

Genetic Factors

Autosomal dominant
- PARK1/PARK4 (SNCA)
- PARK3
- PARK5 (UCH-L1)
- VPS35
- PARK8 (LRRK)
- PARK13 (Omi/H-trA2

Autosomal recessive
- PARK2 (Parkin)
- PARK6 (PINK1)
- PARK7 (DJ-1)
- PARK9 (ATP13A2)
- PARK14 (PLA2G6)
- PARK15 (FBX07

Potential Environmental Factors

- Smoking
- Alcohol use
- BMI
- Diet
- Hypertension

- Pesticides/insecticides
- Fungicides
- Metals
- Organic solvents
- Magnetic fields

FIGURE 2.9. Although the majority of PD cases are sporadic, approximately 10% of cases are due to genetic causes, most notably polymorphisms in SNCA (aka PARK1/PARK4), which is the gene for aSyn. Several environmental factors, as well as being male, have also been suggested to increase one's risk for developing PD (Alafuzoff and Hartikainen, 2017; Delgado-Morales and Esteller, 2017).

BMI: body mass index

Parkinson's Disease Dementia

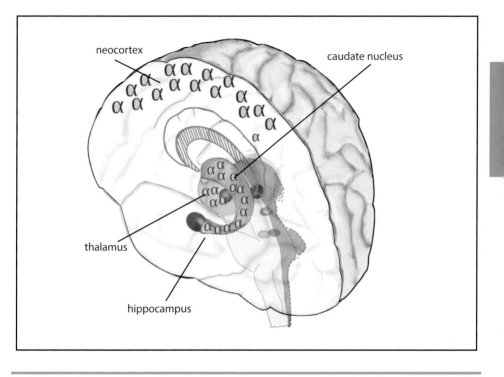

FIGURE 2.10. The majority (~80%) of patients with PD will develop cognitive dysfunction as the disease progresses, with the average time from diagnosis of PD to the onset of dementia being 10 years. Parkinson's disease dementia (PDD) is associated with increased morbidity and ultimately death occurring, on average, 4 years after PDD onset. As with Alzheimer's disease, the harbinger of dementia in Parkinson's disease is often mild cognitive impairment (MCI). Symptoms of PDD include impairments in memory (including recognition), executive dysfunction, deficits in attention, and altered visual perception. The pathological basis for PDD is hypothesized to be neuronal degeneration and atrophy occurring in the thalamus, caudate nucleus, and hippocampus. Lewy body pathology is also often found in neocortical areas; however, the severity of αSyn (as well as amyloid and tau) pathology in limbic regions correlates with the severity of dementia (Foo et al, 2017; Jellinger, 2018; Yang and Yu, 2017; Delgado-Morales and Esteller, 2017).

Parkinson's Disease Dementia Diagnosis

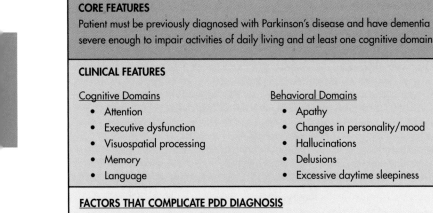

CORE FEATURES
Patient must be previously diagnosed with Parkinson's disease and have dementia severe enough to impair activities of daily living and at least one cognitive domain

CLINICAL FEATURES

Cognitive Domains
- Attention
- Executive dysfunction
- Visuospatial processing
- Memory
- Language

Behavioral Domains
- Apathy
- Changes in personality/mood
- Hallucinations
- Delusions
- Excessive daytime sleepiness

FACTORS THAT COMPLICATE PDD DIAGNOSIS
- Comorbid vascular disease causing cognitive impairment
- Unknown duration of time between motor and cognitive symptom onset

FACTORS THAT MAKE PDD DIAGNOSIS IMPOSSIBLE
- Cognitive/behavioral symptoms occur only in the context of other conditions (e.g., drug intoxication, systemic disease, depression)
- Brain imaging/neurological testing compatible with vascular dementia

FIGURE 2.11. For a diagnosis of probable PDD, the patient must exhibit the core features and deficits in at least two of the four cognitive domains. The presence of behavioral symptoms is supportive of a PDD diagnosis. Features that complicate the diagnosis or make a reliable diagnosis impossible must be absent.

For a diagnosis of possible PDD, the patient must exhibit the core features and deficits in at least one of the four cognitive domains. The presence of behavioral symptoms is supportive of a PDD diagnosis. Features that complicate the diagnosis may be present, but features that make reliable diagnosis impossible must be absent (McKeith et al, 2005; Emre, 2007).

Braak Staging of Lewy Body Pathology

Braak Stage	Lewy Body Pathology
1	Dorsal motor nucleus and/or intermediate reticular zone
2	Caudal raphe nuclei, gigantocellular reticular nucleus, and coeruleus–subcoeruleus complex
3	Midbrain lesions, in particular in the pars compacta of the substantia nigra
4	Prosencephalic lesions, cortical involvement confined to the temporal mesocortex and allocortex
5	High-order sensory association areas of the neocortex and prefrontal neocortex
6	First-order sensory association areas of the neocortex and premotor areas, occasionally mild changes in primary sensory areas and the primary motor field

FIGURE 2.12. Lewy body pathology in Parkinson's disease often follows a defined course as the disease progresses. The pathological progression of Lewy bodies from motor nuclei to other cortical areas is hypothetically related to the clinical progression of Parkinson's disease dementia from motor deficits to psychosis and dementia. As the disease progresses, not only are dopaminergic neurons involved, but serotonergic deficits (note the progression of pathology to the raphe nucleus—the source of serotonergic neurons) may also affect both motor and non-motor presentations in Parkinson's disease (Braak et al, 2003).

Differential Diagnosis: Dementia with Lewy Bodies vs. Parkinson's Disease Dementia

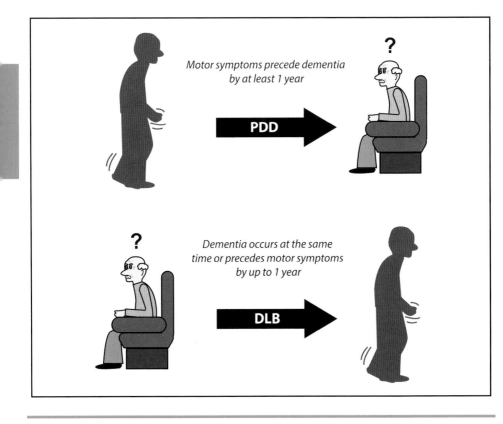

FIGURE 2.13. There is much debate over whether dementia with Lewy bodies (DLB) and Parkinson's disease dementia (PDD) are actually the same disease with slightly different clinical expression and progression, or two distinct diseases. Certainly, PDD and DLB share many pathophysiological and clinical characteristics, and the differential diagnosis between DLB and PDD relies mainly on the onset of motor symptoms vs. the onset of dementia. If motor symptoms precede dementia by 1 year or more, the diagnosis is PDD; however, if dementia occurs at the same time or precedes the onset of parkinsonism, the diagnosis is DLB. Many argue that this "1-year rule" is arbitrary and offers little in terms of treatment guidance (Jellinger, 2018).

Dementia with Lewy Bodies vs. Parkinson's Disease Dementia

Compared to PDD, patients with DLB may have:
More αSyn pathology in temporal and parietal cortices
More Aβ and tau pathology in cortex, striatum, and hippocampus
Neuron loss preferentially in substantia nigra pars compacta
More gray matter cortical atrophy
More white matter hypointensities in temporal lobes
Greater neuroleptic sensitivity
Poorer response to levodopa treatment

FIGURE 2.14. Although there is much debate over the diagnostic utility of DLB vs. PDD, there are several clinical and pathological features that may differ between DLB and PDD. The clinical presentation of each of these LBDs is hypothesized to result from α-synuclein (αSyn), amyloid beta (Aβ), and tau pathology presence, severity, and progression in/through specific brain regions. Dementia with Lewy bodies (DLB) accounts for ~5% of dementia cases and, after the onset of symptoms (typically fluctuating cognitive deficits, visual hallucinations, and REM sleep behavior disorder), the average survival rate is 5–8 years (Jellinger, 2018; Yang and Yu, 2017).

Dementia with Lewy Bodies: Genetics

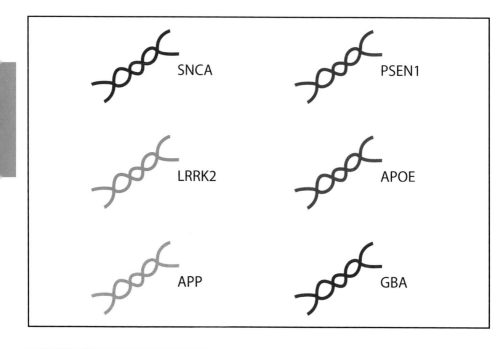

FIGURE 2.15. Although most DLB is sporadic, similar to Alzheimer's disease (AD), there are several genes that convey risk for the development of DLB. Not surprisingly, polymorphisms (more specifically, a triplication) in the gene for a-synuclein (SNCA) have been implicated in both DLB and Parkinson's disease dementia (PDD). Another gene that has been connected with both DLB and PDD is LRRK2, which codes for leucine-rich repeat kinase-2, a protein involved in autophagy regulation, neurite outgrowth, and vesicle trafficking. Interestingly, polymorphisms in genes commonly associated with AD (APP, PSEN1, and APOEε4) have also been implicated in DLB, although this is perhaps not too surprising given the prevalence (up to 80%) of comorbid AD pathology in patients with DLB. Mutations in the gene for glucocerebrosidase (GBA), an enzyme involved in lysosomal storage, have also been found to increase one's risk of developing DLB or PDD (Li et al, 2014; Delgado-Morales and Estelle, 2017; Hinz and Geschwind, 2017).

Dementia with Lewy Bodies: Diagnosis

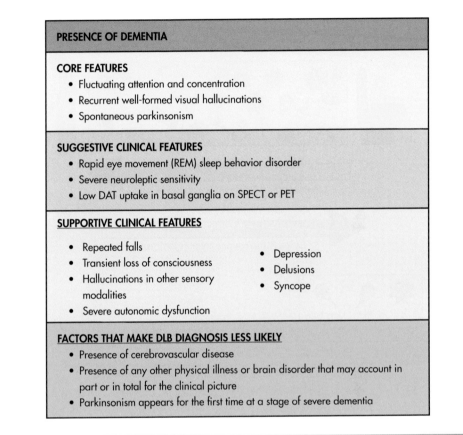

PRESENCE OF DEMENTIA

CORE FEATURES
- Fluctuating attention and concentration
- Recurrent well-formed visual hallucinations
- Spontaneous parkinsonism

SUGGESTIVE CLINICAL FEATURES
- Rapid eye movement (REM) sleep behavior disorder
- Severe neuroleptic sensitivity
- Low DAT uptake in basal ganglia on SPECT or PET

SUPPORTIVE CLINICAL FEATURES
- Repeated falls
- Transient loss of consciousness
- Hallucinations in other sensory modalities
- Severe autonomic dysfunction
- Depression
- Delusions
- Syncope

FACTORS THAT MAKE DLB DIAGNOSIS LESS LIKELY
- Presence of cerebrovascular disease
- Presence of any other physical illness or brain disorder that may account in part or in total for the clinical picture
- Parkinsonism appears for the first time at a stage of severe dementia

FIGURE 2.16. For a diagnosis of probable DLB, the patient must exhibit dementia plus at least two of the core features *or* dementia and only one core feature plus at least one suggestive feature.

For a diagnosis of possible DLB, the patient must exhibit dementia plus either one core feature *or* one suggestive feature (McKeith et al, 2005; Emre, 2007).

PET: positron emission tomography; SPECT: single-photon emission computerized tomography

The Parkinson's–Alzheimer's Disease Spectrum Hypothesis

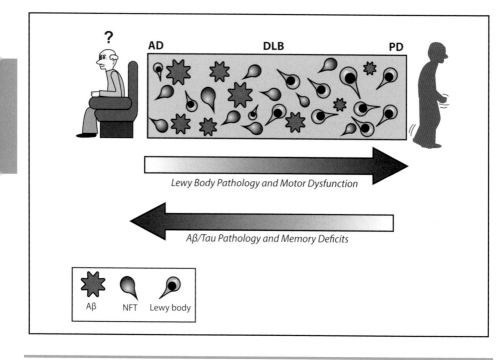

FIGURE 2.17. Although Alzheimer's and Parkinson's diseases have historically been viewed as two distinct entities, the overlap between the disorders has increasingly been recognized. As many as 70% of patients with AD eventually show extrapyramidal and parkinsonian symptoms, and Lewy bodies are seen in ~30% of patients with AD. Likewise, ~50% of patients with PD develop dementia and often have Alzheimer-type pathology. Dementia with Lewy bodies (DLB) shares many neuropsychiatric features with AD as well as many motor features (albeit often less severe) with PD. Due to this overlap in pathology and clinical presentation, some now propose that AD and PD may lie on opposite ends of a spectrum, with DLB falling somewhere between AD and PD. It has been proposed that an individual's neuropsychiatric and physical clinical presentation may be a result of the unique combination of pathological proteins present in the brain as well as the particular brain regions most affected (i.e., more or less AD pathology plus more or less PD pathology combined with a cortical vs. subcortical abundance of pathology) (Jellinger, 2018; Ince et al, 1998; Noe et al, 2004; Anang et al, 2014; Goldman and Holden, 2014; Delgado-Morales and Esteller, 2017).

Differentiating Lewy Body Dementias from Alzheimer's Disease

Compared to AD, patients with DLB may have:
More hypometabolism on FDG-PET
Reduced striatal dopamine transporter (DAT) binding on SPECT or ^{18}fluorodopa PET
Less hippocampal and medial temporal lobe atrophy on MRI
Greater white-matter hyperintensities in occipital lobe on MRI
Better episodic and verbal memory skills
Greater impairments in attention
Memory deficits in retrieval rather than encoding
Memory deficits appearing later in disease course
Early symptoms of sleep disturbances, visual hallucinations, slowness, gait imbalance, or other parkinsonian symptoms
Fluctuating course of cognitive impairment

FIGURE 2.18. As many as 80% of patients with Lewy body dementias (LBDs) have co-occurring Alzheimer's disease (AD) pathology, with only 20% having "pure Lewy body pathology". Although there is significant overlap between Parkinson's disease dementia (PDD) and DLB, the differential diagnosis between DLB and AD is often most difficult due to very similar clinical presentations between AD and DLB, the overlapping pathologies, and the inherent difficulties in eliciting motor symptoms in individuals with dementia. In fact, 2 out of every 3 cases of DLB may be misdiagnosed as AD. However, the accurate differential diagnosis between AD and DLB is important because some treatments currently used in AD may be contraindicated in DLB. There are some key clinical and neuroimaging features that can aid in distinguishing between AD and DLB (Allan et al 2017; Atri, 2016; Karantzoulis and Galvin, 2011; Alzheimer's Association, 2017; Gurnani and Gavett, 2016; Sarro et al, 2017) .

Differentiating Lewy Body Dementias from Alzheimer's Disease: Finger Displacement

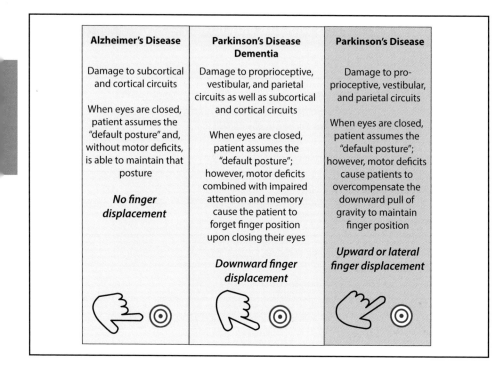

Alzheimer's Disease	Parkinson's Disease Dementia	Parkinson's Disease
Damage to subcortical and cortical circuits	Damage to proprioceptive, vestibular, and parietal circuits as well as subcortical and cortical circuits	Damage to proprioceptive, vestibular, and parietal circuits
When eyes are closed, patient assumes the "default posture" and, without motor deficits, is able to maintain that posture	When eyes are closed, patient assumes the "default posture"; however, motor deficits combined with impaired attention and memory cause the patient to forget finger position upon closing their eyes	When eyes are closed, patient assumes the "default posture"; however, motor deficits cause patients to overcompensate the downward pull of gravity to maintain finger position
No finger displacement	*Downward finger displacement*	*Upward or lateral finger displacement*

FIGURE 2.19. Recent data indicate that PDD can be distinguished from AD (as well as Parkinson's disease without dementia) using a simple, in-office procedure that costs relatively little time and money. The test involves having a patient point their index finger at a fixed target for 15 seconds with eyes open, then 15 seconds with eyes closed, and has been shown to accurately differentiate patients as having either PDD or AD based solely on this simple, non-invasive finger displacement test. Patients with AD typically do not show any finger displacement whereas patients with PD typically exhibit an upward or lateral finger displacement. Patients with PDD, who hypothetically have neuropathological features in common with both AD and PD, tend to have downward finger displacement when their eyes are closed. Discrepancies in finger displacement between PD, PDD, and AD are hypothetically due to the different pathological processes that tax various brain regions. Future studies may help utilize the finger displacement test as a means for aiding in the differential diagnosis between DLB and AD or DLB and PD (Lieberman et al, 2018).

Assessment Tools for Lewy Body Dementias

	LBCRS	UPDRS	NMSS
Assesses:	Likelihood that Lewy body pathology is contributing to cognitive dysfunction	Both motor and non-motor symptoms of PD	Non-motor symptoms of PD
Questions Covering:	• Motor symptoms • Non-motor symptoms	• Mentation, behavior, and mood • Activities of daily living • Motor examination • Complications of therapy	• Cardiovascular function • Sleep/fatigue • Mood/cognition • Perceptual problems/ hallucinations • Attention/memory • Gastrointestinal function • Urinary function • Sexual function
# of Questions	10	42	30

FIGURE 2.20. Several rating scales and assessment tools have been developed to aid in measurement of symptom severity and differential diagnosis in Lewy body dementias (LBDs), including the Lewy Body Composite Risk Score (LBCRS), the Unified Parkinson's Disease Rating Scale (UPDRS), and the Non-Motor Symptom Assessment Scale for Parkinson's Disease (NMSS) (Thomas et al, 2017b; Yang and Yu, 2017; Goetz et al, 2008; Galvin, 2015).

Treatment of Lewy Body Dementias

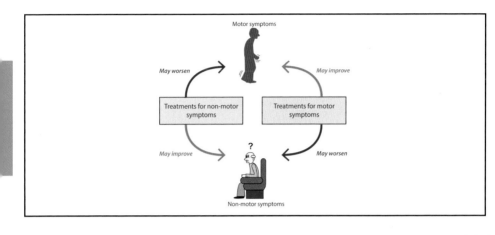

FIGURE 2.21. Unfortunately, as with AD, there is no disease-modifying treatment yet available for DLB or PDD. L-dopa and dopamine agonists are often used to treat the motor symptoms in LBDs; however, these agents may, in fact, worsen psychosis (and potentially dementia) and are generally less effective for motor symptoms in DLB compared to PD. While memantine and cholinesterase inhibitors may have some efficacy in reducing psychotic symptoms in LBDs, their use is limited in LBDs. In addition to a Black Box warning regarding the increased risk of mortality associated with antipsychotic use in all elderly patients with dementia, patients with DLB may be particularly sensitive to the development of extrapyramidal symptoms (EPS) and mortality associated with antipsychotics. Pimavanserin, a novel antipsychotic that acts as a 5HT2A antagonist with no effects on dopamine D2 receptors, is approved for the treatment of psychosis in PD (and hypothetically may be useful for psychosis in DLB as well) and does not appear to worsen motor symptoms. Pimavanserin is also being investigated for its use in psychosis associated with AD with some promising preliminary results. Pimavanserin should likely be considered the first line in the treatment of psychosis associated with PD (and perhaps DLB); however, in the event that an older antipsychotic must be used, quetiapine or clozapine would be recommended above other atypical antipsychotics due to their relatively lessened risk of EPS. Future treatments may one day include agents that inhibit αSyn aggregation or increase αSyn degradation and, given the overlap between AD and LBD pathologies, AD disease-modifying treatments currently being investigated for AD may also potentially have some utility in treating LBDs (Preuss et al, 2016; Yang and Yu, 2017; Alafuzoff and Hartikainen, 2017; Jellinger, 2018; Stahl, 2016).

Multiple System Atrophy

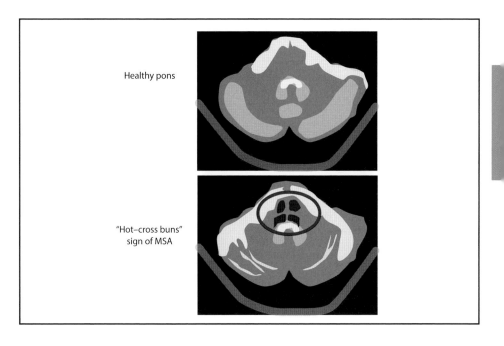

Healthy pons

"Hot–cross buns" sign of MSA

FIGURE 2.22. Multiple system atrophy (MSA) is another synucleinopathy. However, unlike in the Lewy body dementias (LBDs), in MSA, αSyn accumulates not in the neuronal soma (resulting in the characteristic Lewy bodies seen in PDD and LBD), but rather the αSyn aggregation in MSA occurs in glial cells, resulting in characteristic pathological lesions called oligodendroglial cytoplasmic inclusions. The clinical presentation of MSA includes parkinsonism, cerebellar ataxia (such as difficulties with speech, ocular movements, and swallowing), autonomic failure, motor weakness, cognitive decline, and eventually, dementia. Although the definitive diagnosis of MSA can only be made postmortem, designation MSA-C is used to denote cases where cerebellar symptoms are the dominant clinical presentation, and MSA-P is the designation when parkinsonism is the prevailing symptom. Typically in MSA, atrophy occurs in the cerebellum, pons, inferior olives, locus coeruleus, and striatum. In fact, a characteristic hallmark seen on MRI in patients with MSA-C includes a so-called "hot–cross bun" sign due to atrophy in the pons. Unfortunately, currently available treatments are not disease-modifying and focus mostly on ameliorating autonomic symptoms (Alafuzoff and Hartikainen, 2017; Deutschlander et al, 2018; Meyer et al, 2017).

Unified Multiple System Atrophy Rating Scale

PART 1. Historical Review
- Speech
- Swallowing
- Handwriting
- Cutting food/ handling utensils
- Dressing
- Hygiene
- Walking
- Falling
- Orthostatic symptoms
- Urinary function
- Sexual function
- Bowel function

PART 2. Motor Examination
- Facial expression
- Speech
- Ocular motor function
- Resting tremor
- Action tremor
- Increased tone
- Rapid alternating hand movements
- Finger taps
- Leg agility
- Heel–knee–shin test
- Arising from chair
- Posture
- Body sway
- Gait

PART 3. Autonomic Examination
- Systolic blood pressure
- Diastolic blood pressure
- Heart rate
- Orthostatic symptoms

PART 4. Global Disability
- Rated from 1 (completely independent) to 5 (completely dependent)

FIGURE 2.23. Clinical assessment of patients with MSA can be carried out using the Unified MSA Rating Scale, a 4-part scale designed to measure the severity of functional disability, motor deficits, autonomic deficits, and global functioning (Wenning et al, 2004).

REM Sleep Behavior Disorder in Alpha-Synucleinopathies

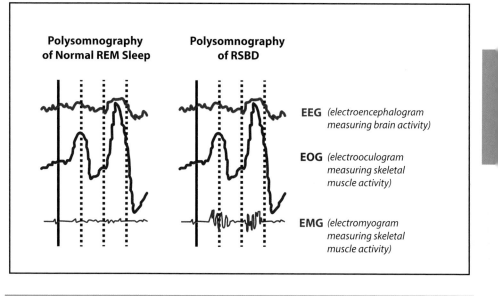

Polysomnography of Normal REM Sleep

Polysomnography of RSBD

EEG *(electroencephalogram measuring brain activity)*

EOG *(electrooculogram measuring skeletal muscle activity)*

EMG *(electromyogram measuring skeletal muscle activity)*

FIGURE 2.24. Typically, during rapid eye movement (REM) sleep (a period of sleep in which we dream), an individual exhibits brain wave patterns on polysomnography that are similar to those seen during periods of wakefulness with ocular motor activity but an absence of skeletal muscle activity (i.e., atonia). In patients with REM sleep behavior disorder (RSBD), there is a lack of atonia during REM sleep which causes patients to "act out" their dreams, potentially leading to injury to themselves and others. Although RSBD is quite rare in the general population (<1%), it is actually quite common (50% or more) in patients with α-synucleinopathies (including PD, LBD, and MSA) and is hypothesized to relate to pathology and neurodegeneration in the pedunculopontine nucleus and disinhibition of spinal and brainstem motor neurons. Not only is RSBD a common symptom seen in LBDs and MSA, it often manifests years (even decades) before the onset of motor symptoms and may be a prodromal symptom of an impending α-synuclein-related motor and cognitive dysfunction; indeed, more than 80% of individuals with RBSD are eventually identified as having a synucleinopathy. Unfortunately, antidepressants, which are often used to treat neuropsychiatric symptoms in LBDs and MSA, may exacerbate RSBD. Clonazepam (0.5–2mg/day) and melatonin (3–8mg/day) taken before bedtime have the most evidence of efficacy for RSBD, with melatonin having a better safety profile compared to clonazepam (Bassetti and Bargiotas, 2018; Johnson and Westlake, 2017).

Frontotemporal Lobar Degeneration and Tauopathies

Frontotemporal lobar degeneration (FTLD) is an umbrella term describing a group of different disorders with varying clinical presentations, genetics, and pathophysiology. Although not all FTLD disorders have pathological tau as the neurobiological substrate for clinical symptoms, all FTLD disorders share some cognitive and/or motor features. Frontotemporal dementia (FTD), progressive supranuclear palsy (PSP), corticobasal degeneration (CBD), argyrophilic grain disease (AGD), and amyotrophic lateral sclerosis (ALS) can all be classified as types of FTLD. As we will see in this chapter, there is significant overlap among the assorted types of FTLD disorders as well as shared clinical, genetic, and pathological characteristics among tauopathies and with the other dementias previously discussed (Alzheimer's disease and α-synucleinopathies). For strategies to ameliorate some of the secondary behavioral symptoms often associated with FTLD and other dementias, the reader is directed to Chapter 5 (Park et al, 2017; Karantzoulis and Galvin, 2011; Atri, 2016).

FTLD in Relation to Other Dementias: Genes

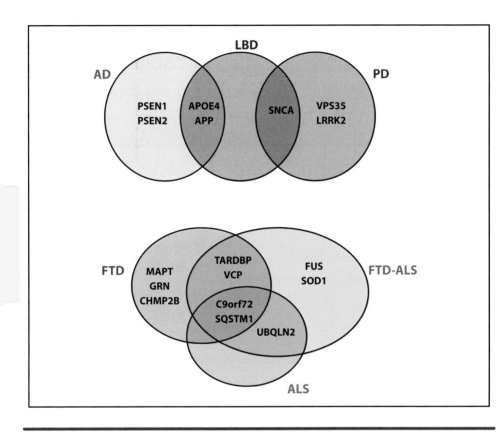

FIGURE 3.1. Although most cases of FTLD are sporadic, there are several genetic mutations that can give rise to familial FTLD. There is also significant overlap, in terms of genetic predisposition among AD, LBD, and FTLDs such as FTD and ALS. The shared genetic links among these different dementias likely contribute to much of the overlap in pathophysiology and symptoms (Hinz and Geschwind, 2017).

FTLD in Relation to Other Dementias: Pathological Proteins

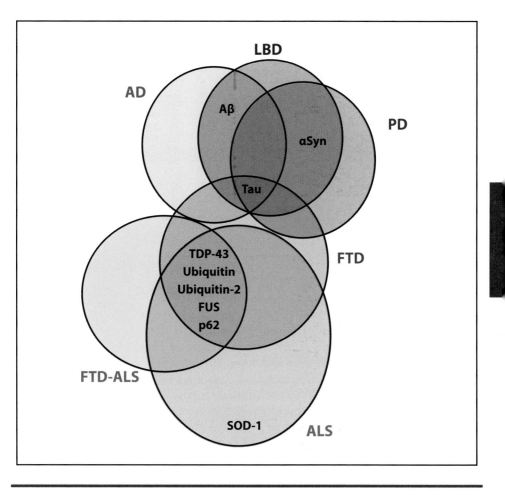

FIGURE 3.2. AD, LBD, FTD, and ALS also have significant overlap in terms of the pathological proteins that may be present in various brain regions and likely contribute to neurodegeneration and dementia (Hinz and Geschwind, 2017).

FTLD: Genetics and Pathology

	FTLD-Tau+	FTLD-TDP+	FTLD-FET+
% of FTLD	45%	50%	5%
Associated with mutations in…	• MAPT	• TARDBP • C9orf72 • GRN	• FUS
Pathological proteins include…	• pTau	• TDP-43 • Ubiquitin • p62	• FUS • EWSR1 • TAF15
May present as…	• bvFTD • FTDP-17 • Pick's disease • AGD • PSP	• bvFTD • nfvPPA • PSP • CBD • MND	• ALS • Atypical FTLD • BIBD • NIFID

FIGURE 3.3. Neuropathologically, frontotemporal lobar degeneration (FTLD) may be categorized as Tau+ or Tau– depending on the presence of hyperphosphorylated tau protein (pTau); Tau– cases may be further categorized as TDP-43+ or TDP-43– depending on the presence of transactive response DNA binding protein of 43 kDA (TDP-43; TARDBP); another classification includes FET+ or FET– (where FET denotes a family of proteins including fused in sarcoma [FUS], Ewing's sarcoma protein [EWSR1], and TATA-binding protein-associated factor 15 [TAF15]). Overall, the genetics and pathology of FTLD are relatively complex compared to the disorders discussed so far. Mutations in progranulin (GRN) and tau (MAPT), as well as a hexanucleotide repeat in chromosome 9 open reading frame (C9orf72), have been most notably associated with different FTLD types. Mutations in TARDBP, valosin-containing protein (VCP), sequestosome 1 (SQSTM1), superoxide dismutase 1 (SOD1), ubiquilin 2 (UBQL2), and chromatin-modifying 2B (CHMP2B) have also less commonly been causative of FTLD (Park et al, 2017; Deutschlander et al, 2018; Ling, 2016; Weishaupt et al, 2016; Dugger and Dickson, 2017; Hasegawa et al, 2017; Olszewska et al, 2016; Hinz and Geschwind, 2017).

AGD: argyrophilic grain disease; ALS: amyotrophic lateral sclerosis; BIBD: basophilic inclusion body disease; bvFTD: behavioral variant frontotemporal dementia; CBD: corticobasal degeneration; FTDP-17: frontotemporal dementia and parkinsonism linked to chromosome 17; MND: motor neuron disease; NIFID: neuronal intermediate filament- and α-internexin-positive inclusions; nfvPPA: non-fluent variant primary progressive aphasia; PSP: progressive supranuclear palsy

Microtubule-Associated Protein Tau (MAPT)

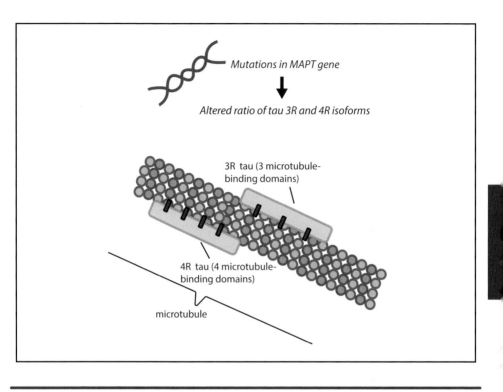

Mutations in MAPT gene

Altered ratio of tau 3R and 4R isoforms

3R tau (3 microtubule-binding domains)

4R tau (4 microtubule-binding domains)

microtubule

FIGURE 3.4. Although aggregation of phosphorylated tau (pTau) into neurofibrillary tangles (NFTs) is a hallmark feature of Alzheimer's disease (AD), the gene coding for the tau protein (microtubule-associated protein tau; MAPT) is actually not associated with AD. Rather, MAPT mutations are associated with several forms of FTLD (including frontotemporal dementia with parkinsonism linked to chromosome 17 (FTDP-17), behavioral variant FTD (bvFTD), and progressive supranuclear palsy (PSP). Each of these disorders may have aggregation and progression of tau pathology; however, the specific distribution of pathological tau differs slightly for each specific disorder, bringing about an array of clinical symptomatology. Greater than 40 pathological mutations in MAPT have been discovered and account for ~50% of all FTLD cases. Typically, these mutations change the ratio of tau 3R and 4R isoforms, leading to an accumulation of pathological tau (Mackenzie and Neumann, 2016; Hinz and Geschwind, 2017; Delgado-Morales and Esteller, 2017).

Progranulin (GRN)

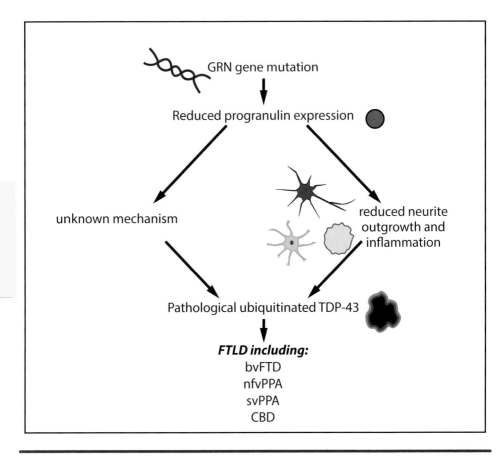

FIGURE 3.5. The GRN gene codes for progranulin, a glycoprotein that is potentially involved in neurotrophic and anti-inflammatory processes. Mutations in GRN (present in as many as 11% of individuals with FTLD) lead to the deficient production of progranulin and subsequent build-up of pathological ubiquitinated TDP-43; however, the exact mechanism by which deficient progranulin levels lead to pathological TDP-43 is unclear. As with pathological tau protein, the location and progression of TDP-43 pathology (as well as specific FTD-43 morphology) may differ between specific FTLD disorders (Gass et al, 2012; Hinz and Geschwind, 2017).

Chromosome 9 Open Reading Frame 72 (C9orf72)

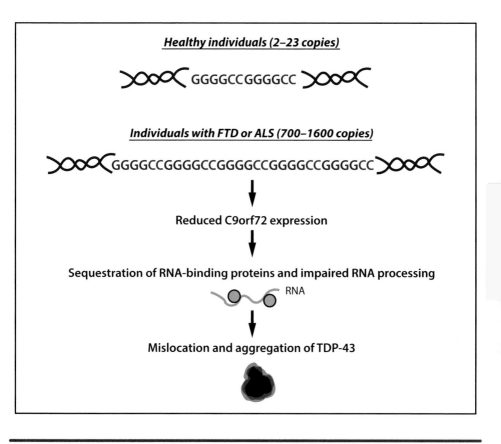

FIGURE 3.6. The chromosome 9 open reading frame 72 (C9orf72) is a hexanucleotide repeat (GGGGCC) in a non-coding region of chromosome 9. Healthy individuals typically have ~2–23 copies of this hexanucleotide whereas patients with frontotemporal dementia (FTD) amyotrophic lateral sclerosis (ALS) may have 700–1600 copies. This C9orf72 repeat expansion is the most common genetic cause of both FTD and ALS. Through an as-yet unelucidated mechanism, C9orf72 repeat expansion induces a mislocation and aggregation of TDP-43 in cortical neurons (FTD), motor neurons (ALS) or both (FTD-ALS). It is hypothesized that the C9orf72 repeat expansion causes a reduced production of C9orf72 and leads to sequestration of RNA-binding proteins and subsequent impairments in RNA processing (Todd and Petrucelli, 2016; Kumar et al, 2017).

Valosin-Containing Protein (VCP)

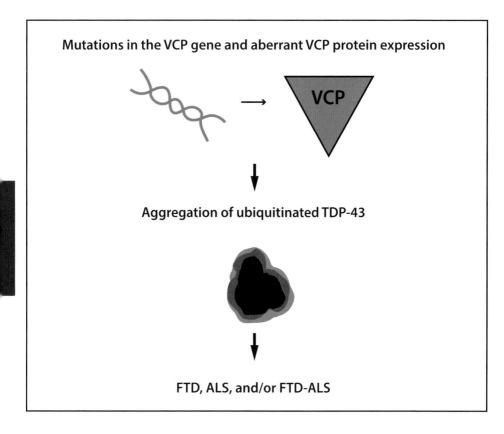

Mutations in the VCP gene and aberrant VCP protein expression

VCP

Aggregation of ubiquitinated TDP-43

FTD, ALS, and/or FTD-ALS

FIGURE 3.7. Valosin-containing protein (VCP) is hypothesized to be involved in a number of cellular processes, including membrane fusion, transcription activation, nuclear envelope reconstruction, DNA repair, mitosis and cell cycle control, apoptosis, and degradation of proteins. In addition to being associated with inclusion body myositis with Paget's disease (a rare bone and muscle disorder), mutations in the VCP gene can also (uncommonly) cause a form of FTLD-TDP, including amyotrophic lateral sclerosis (ALS) and frontotemporal dementia (FTD) and the combined pathological presentation of combined ALS-FTD. Through an unknown mechanism, VCP mutations can lead to accumulation of ubiquitinated TDP-43 protein in ALS and FTD (Mackenzie and Neumann, 2016; Nalbandian et al, 2011).

Transactive Response Element-Binding Protein 43 (TDP-43)

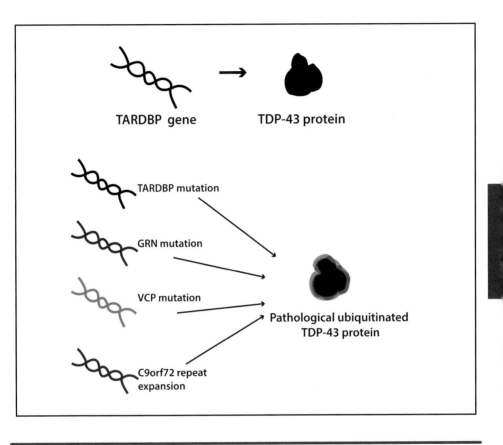

TARDBP gene → TDP-43 protein

TARDBP mutation

GRN mutation

VCP mutation

C9orf72 repeat expansion

Pathological ubiquitinated TDP-43 protein

FIGURE 3.8. The gene TARDBP codes for the protein transactive response element-binding protein 43 (TDP-43), a ribonucleoprotein involved in RNA splicing and stability, apoptosis, and cell division. Although mutations in TARDBP are rare, pathological, ubiquitinated TDP-43 protein is found in many FTLD disorders, sometimes as a consequence of mutations in the GRN (progranulin) or VCP (valosin-containing protein) genes or as a result of a hexanucleotide repeat expansion in chromosome 9 open reading frame 72 (C9orf72). TDP-43 pathology can be categorized into four types (Types A–D) based on its morphology and location and may also be found in non-FTLD disorders including AD and DLBs (Arai, 2014; Hinz and Geschwind, 2017; Dugger and Dickson, 2017; Deutschlander et al, 2018; Mackenzie and Neumann, 2016; Mackenzie et al, 2011; Forman et al, 2007).

TDP-43 Type A

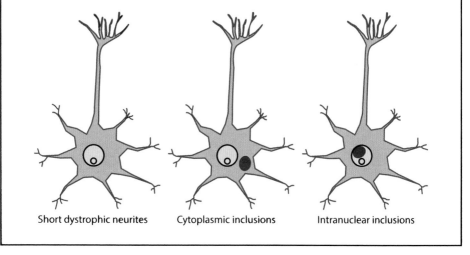

TYPE A
- Most common
- Compact neuronal cytoplasmic inclusions
- Short dystrophic cortical neurites
- Neuronal intranuclear inclusions
- Predominantly cortical layer 2 pathology
- Sparing of hippocampal neurites
- Associated with GRN mutations and C9orf72 repeat expansion
- Often found in bvFTD and nfvPPA

Short dystrophic neurites   Cytoplasmic inclusions   Intranuclear inclusions

FIGURE 3.9. Type A TDP-43 pathology is the most common subtype, accounting for ~41% of FTD-TDP cases. Pathological inclusions in Type A include all three morphological aggregates of TDP-43: dystrophic neurites, neuronal cytoplasmic inclusions, and neuronal intranuclear inclusions (Arai, 2014; Mackenzie and Neumann, 2016; Mackenzie et al, 2011; Forman et al, 2007).

TDP-43 Type B

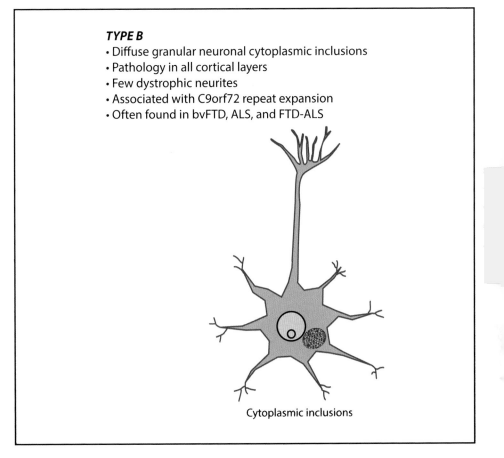

TYPE B
- Diffuse granular neuronal cytoplasmic inclusions
- Pathology in all cortical layers
- Few dystrophic neurites
- Associated with C9orf72 repeat expansion
- Often found in bvFTD, ALS, and FTD-ALS

Cytoplasmic inclusions

FIGURE 3.10. Type B TDP-43 pathology is the second most common form and is evidenced in ~34% of patients with FTLD-TDP. Type B TDP-43 pathology is often associated with FTLD with comorbid motor neuron disease features (such as amyotrophic lateral sclerosis; ALS), likely as a result of its propensity to accumulate in motor areas as well as cortical and subcortical regions. Type B TDP-43 pathology typically consists of primarily neuronal cytoplasmic inclusions that are often more granular and less compact than those seen in Type A (Arai, 2014; Mackenzie and Neumann, 2016; Mackenzie et al, 2011; Forman et al, 2007).

TDP-43 Type C

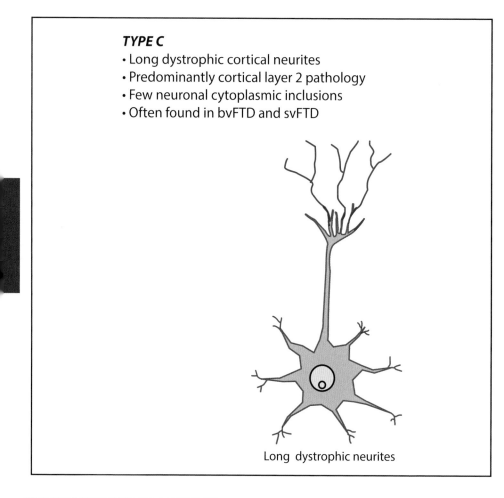

TYPE C
- Long dystrophic cortical neurites
- Predominantly cortical layer 2 pathology
- Few neuronal cytoplasmic inclusions
- Often found in bvFTD and svFTD

Long dystrophic neurites

FIGURE 3.11. Type C TDP-43 pathology is less common than either Type A or B and accounts for ~17% of FTLD-TDP cases. Dystrophic neurites are the primary pathological feature of Type C TDP-43 pathology and these neurites are often longer than those seen in either Type A or Type D (Arai, 2014; Mackenzie and Neumann, 2016; Mackenzie et al, 2011; Forman et al, 2007).

TDP-43 Type D

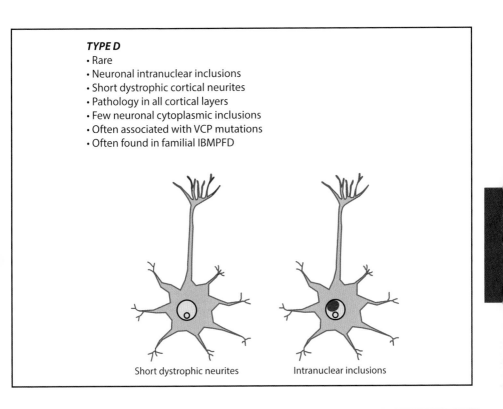

TYPE D
- Rare
- Neuronal intranuclear inclusions
- Short dystrophic cortical neurites
- Pathology in all cortical layers
- Few neuronal cytoplasmic inclusions
- Often associated with VCP mutations
- Often found in familial IBMPFD

Short dystrophic neurites   Intranuclear inclusions

FIGURE 3.12. Type D is the most rare pathological characterization of TDP-43 and is more commonly associated with a bone and muscle disorder called inclusion body myositis with Paget's disease of bone and FTD (IBMPFD) than with pure FTD subtypes (Arai, 2014; Mackenzie and Neumann, 2016; Mackenzie et al, 2011; Forman et al, 2007).

Frontotemporal Dementia

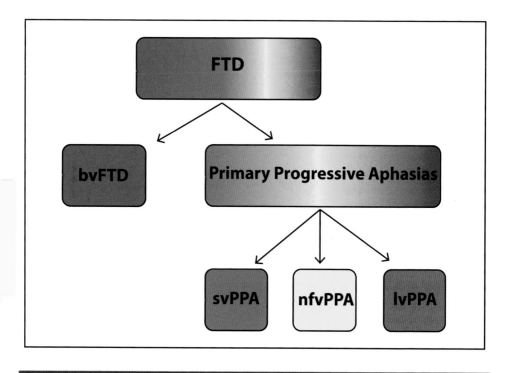

FIGURE 3.13. Frontotemporal dementia (FTD) is the 3rd most common form of dementia, with a worldwide prevalence of 3–26% in individuals aged 65 years and older and an average age-of-onset of 50–65 years. FTD is divided into 4 subtypes: behavioral variant FTD (bvFTD), semantic variant primary progressive aphasia (svPPA), and non-fluent variant primary progressive aphasia (nfvPPA), and logopenic variant primary progressive aphasia (lvPPA) depending on the clinical presentation. Pathologically, FTD typically begins with a loss of cortical and basal ganglia neurons as well as gliosis and neurovascular changes predominantly in one hemisphere; however, as the disease progresses, atrophy may become bilateral and extend to additional brain regions. The diagnosis of FTD can be somewhat complex as clinical presentation and pathology often overlap with those of other FTLD disorders (including PSP, CBD, and motor neuron diseases such as ALS) and many patients exhibit parkinsonian-like features. FTD can often be differentiated from AD by the absence of Aβ CSF or PET imaging biomarkers (Hinz and Geschwind, 2017; Delgado-Morales and Esteller, 2017; Gordon et al, 2016; Deutschlander et al, 2018).

Behavioral Variant Frontotemporal Dementia (bvFTD)

Clinical presentation

- Progressive personality changes
  - Disinhibition
  - Apathy
  - Loss of sympathy/empathy
- Hyperorality
- Perseverative/compulsive behaviors
- Cognitive deficits
- Cued memory and visuospatial abilities spared

Pathological presentation

- Atrophy in:
  - PFC
  - Insula
  - Anterior cingulate
  - Striatum
  - Thalamus
- Non-dominant hemisphere more affected

FIGURE 3.14. Behavioral variant FTD (bvFTD), the most common of the FTD subtypes, usually presents with gradual and progressive personality changes (such as disinhibition, apathy, and loss of sympathy and empathy), hyperorality, and perseverative or compulsive behaviors, and eventually, cognitive deficits with a general sparing of visuospatial abilities. Patients with bvFTD are often unaware of their inappropriate behaviors, and contrary to patients with AD, do not typically have rapid memory loss and may do fairly well in memory tasks if provided cues. Pathologically, bvFTD is characterized by frontal and anterior temporal cortex atrophy, particularly the prefrontal cortex (PFC), insula, anterior cingulate, striatum, and thalamus, with the non-dominant hemisphere typically more affected (Deutschlander et al, 2018; Karantzoulis and Galvin, 2011; Gordon et al, 2016; Hinz and Geschwind, 2017; Mallik et al, 2017; McCarter et al, 2016).

Diagnosing bvFTD

Possible bvFTD

At least 3 of the following:

- Disinhibition
- Apathy
- Loss of sympathy or empathy
- Perseverative or compulsive behavior
- Hyperorality
- Executive dysfunction

Probable bvFTD

- Possible bvFTD clinical evidence
- Neuroimaging evidence of frontal and/or temporal lobe atrophy

Definitive bvFTD

- Possible bvFTD clinical evidence
- Histopathological confirmation of pathology or presence of bvFTD-related mutation

FIGURE 3.15. As with most dementias, the certainty of a diagnosis of bvFTD is increased when biomarker and/or genetic evidence support the clinical presentation, with an absolute diagnosis of bvFTD only achievable postmortem (McCarter et al, 2016).

Primary Progressive Aphasia (PPA)

	bvFTD	PPA
Affected Hemisphere	Non-dominant	Dominant
Behavioral Disturbances	More severe	Less severe
Sleep Disturbances	Less severe	More severe
Language Deficits	Less severe	More severe

FIGURE 3.16. The defining characteristic of primary progressive aphasia (PPA) is a deficit in language with impairment in activities of daily living. PPA can be further classified as semantic variant PPA, non-fluent variant PPA, or logopenic variant PPA based on the specific types of language deficits that predominate the clinical picture. In contrast to bvFTD, pathology in the PPAs typically occurs in the dominant hemisphere, behavioral disturbances may be less evident, and sleep disturbances may be more prominent (Landin-Romero et al, 2016; Gordon et al, 2016; Torrisi et al, 2017; Deutschlander et al, 2018; Karantzoulis et al, 2011; McCarter et al, 2016).

Semantic Variant PPA (svPPA)

Typical Features of svPPA
- Type C TDP-43 pathology
- Anterior and inferior temporal lobe atrophy in dominant hemisphere
- Impairments in:
  - *confrontation naming*
  - *single-word comprehension*
  - *object knowledge*
- Dyslexia
- Dysgraphia
- Logorrhea

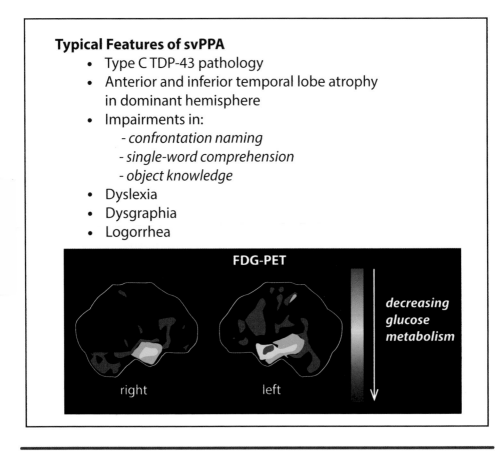

FIGURE 3.17. Patients with semantic variant PPA (svPPA) show impairments in confrontation naming and single-word comprehension, as well as possible impairments in object knowledge and dyslexia or dysgraphia. Patients with svPPA often have speech that is logorrheic—fluent but empty of meaning. As the disease progresses, patients may become almost mute, with only a limited repertoire of stereotypic phrases and no word comprehension. In contrast to AD, episodic memory is relatively spared in svPPA. Pathologically, patients with svPPA show asymmetric anterior and inferior temporal lobe atrophy most often associated with Type C TDP-43 pathology (Landin-Romero et al, 2016; Deutschlander et al, 2018; Karantzoulis and Galvin, 2011; Gordon et al, 2016).

Non-Fluent Variant PPA (nfvPPA)

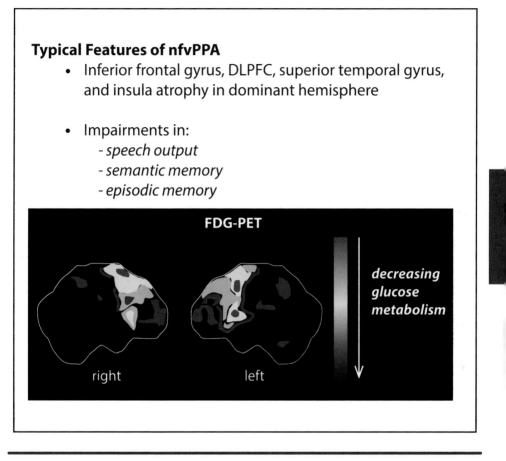

Typical Features of nfvPPA
- Inferior frontal gyrus, DLPFC, superior temporal gyrus, and insula atrophy in dominant hemisphere

- Impairments in:
  - *speech output*
  - *semantic memory*
  - *episodic memory*

FDG-PET

right   left

decreasing glucose metabolism

FIGURE 3.18. In addition to exhibiting episodic memory deficits similar to patients with AD, patients with non-fluent variant PPA (nfvPPA) present with severe deficits in speech output and semantic memory loss. Pathologically, patients with nfvPPA typically show atrophy of the inferior frontal gyrus, dorsolateral prefrontal cortex (DLPFC), superior temporal gyrus, and insula, particularly in the dominant hemisphere (Deutschlander et al, 2018; Gordon et al, 2016).

Logopenic Variant PPA (lvPPA)

Typical Features of lvPPA
- Temporoparietal and cingulate cortical atrophy in dominant hemisphere

- Impairments in:
  - *sentence processing/repetition*
  - *naming of everyday objects*
  - *word finding*

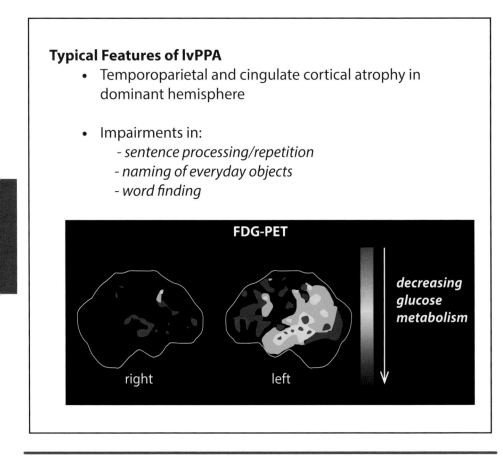

FIGURE 3.19. Logopenic variant PPA (lvPPA) is characterized by prolonged word-finding pauses, anomia (impaired naming of everyday objects), and impaired sentence processing. Pathologically, atrophy in lvPPA tends to be more posterior than that seen in svPPA or nfvPPA and typically involves temporoparietal and cingulate cortices in the dominant hemisphere (Deutschlander et al, 2018; Gordon et al, 2016).

Frontotemporal Dementia with Parkinsonism Linked to Chromosome 17 (FTDP-17)

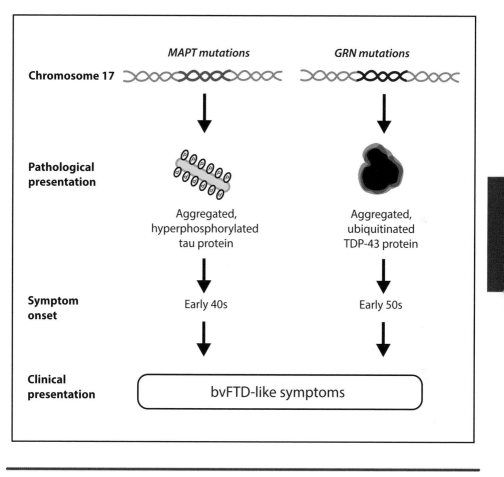

FIGURE 3.20. Frontotemporal dementia linked to parkinsonism on chromosome 17 (FTDP-17) typically presents with behavioral variant frontotemporal dementia (bv-FTD)-like symptoms and is due to mutations on MAPT or GRN genes (both of which are located on chromosome 17). Although both MAPT and GRN mutations can lead to FTDP-17, the age of onset and pathological progression differs; mutations in MAPT lead to FTDP-17 with an age-of-onset in the early 40s and present with tau pathology whereas mutations in GRN lead to FTDP-17 with an age-of-onset in the early 50s and present with TDP-43 pathology (Deutschlander et al, 2018).

Pick's Disease

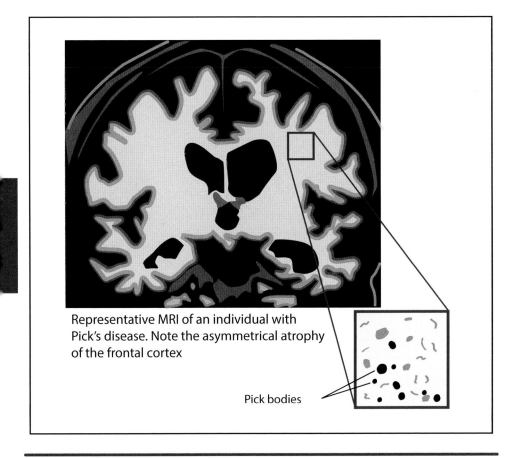

Representative MRI of an individual with Pick's disease. Note the asymmetrical atrophy of the frontal cortex

Pick bodies

FIGURE 3.21. Pick's disease is a rare disorder denoting a type of FTLD that typically presents as bvFTD (personality changes) or nfvPPA (language disturbances, usually without symptoms of parkinsonism). Pathologically, intracytoplasmic "Pick bodies" composed of hyperphosphorylated 3R tau are found asymmetrically in frontal and temporal cortices as well as amygdala, hippocampus, substantia nigra, striatum, and locus coeruleus. Unlike the flame-shaped neurofibrillary tangles that represent accumulated hyperphosphorylated tau in AD, Pick bodies tend to be round and lend a balloon-like structure to cells (i.e., "Pick cells") (Mackenzie and Neumann, 2016; Dugger and Dickson, 2017; Deutschlander et al, 2018; Harper et al, 2014).

Amyotrophic Lateral Sclerosis

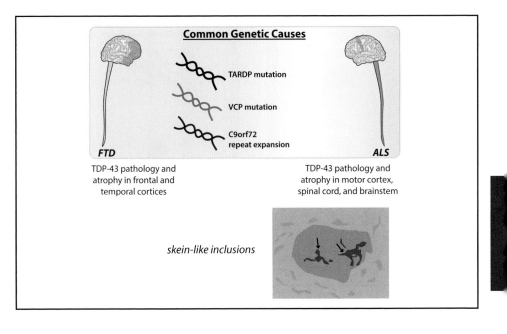

FIGURE 3.22. Amyotrophic lateral sclerosis (ALS), also called Lou Gehrig's disease, is a neurodegenerative motor neuron disease with an incidence of 1–3 individuals in 100,000. ALS is characterized by a progressive weakening of voluntary muscles and muscle atrophy with typical onset around 60–70 years of age. Muscle weakness typically starts with an upper limb, and as ALS symptoms progress, a significant portion of patients develop dementia that is similar to frontotemporal dementia (FTD). Pathologically, ALS is often associated with TDP-43 deposits as skein-like inclusions and atrophy in the motor cortex, spinal cord, and brainstem (underlying motor symptoms) and Type B TDP-43 pathology and atrophy in temporal and frontal lobes (leading to dementia). This pathology outside of motor systems is hypothesized to result in the comorbid FTD-like clinical presentation that often accompanies ALS; 15% of patients with FTD are eventually diagnosed with comorbid ALS. The genetic, pathological, and clinical overlap between ALS and FTD (termed ALS-FTD when co-occurring) also suggests that ALS and motor neuron disease (such as ALS) lie along a continuum rather than representing two completely distinct disorders (Dugger and Dickson, 2016; Weishaupt et al, 2016; Hinz and Geschwind, 2017; Arai, 2014).

Progressive Supranuclear Palsy

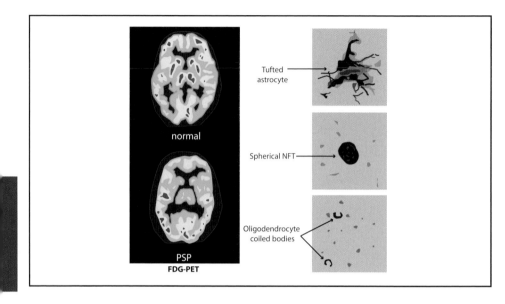

FIGURE 3.23. Progressive supranuclear palsy (PSP) is a tauopathy that usually presents with dysfunction in both movement and cognition. Initially, patients (usually in the 5th or 6th decade of life) complain of symptoms such as blurred vision, dizziness, falls, and fatigue accompanied by apathy, depression, and irritability. Early in the disease course, parkinsonian symptoms and vertical gaze palsy develop, often followed by worsening cognition and bvFTD- or nfvPPA-like dementia (including impaired mental manipulation and problems with recall memory). Histopathological examination reveals accumulation of 4R tau in neurons (as spherical neurofibrillary tangles most notably in subcortical regions), oligodendrocytes (as coiled bodies in white matter), and astrocytes (commonly identified as "tufted astrocytes" most frequently in the motor cortex and neostriatum) associated with severe midbrain atrophy. FDG-PET reveals hypometabolism in anterior cingulate gyrus (leading to vertical gaze palsy), thalamus (causing unexplained falls), midbrain (underlying gait freezing), and dorsolateral frontal lobe (contributing to non-fluent aphasia). Most cases of PSP are sporadic; however, polymorphisms in the MAPT gene have been shown to contribute to increasing risk of PSP (Eusebio et al, 2016; Ling, 2016; Dugger and Dickson, 2017; Mackenzie and Neumann, 2016; Boxer et al, 2017; Deutschlander et al, 2018; Liscic et al, 2013; Meyer et al, 2017).

Progressive Supranuclear Palsy Subtypes

PSP-RS
- Vertical gaze palsy
- Postural instability and falls
- Axial rigidity
- Early cognitive decline
- Early frontal behavioral dysfunction

PSP-P
- Early features of parkinsonism
- Asymmetric onset of tremors
- Bradykinesia
- Limb rigidity
- Moderate response to levodopa

PSP-SL
- Predominant speech or language disorder
- Early cognitive decline
- Early frontal behavioral dysfunction
- Motor features develop later in disease course

PSP-CBS
- Progressive limb rigidity
- Apraxia
- Cortical sensory loss
- Alien limb phenomenon
- Bradykinesia

PSP-F
- Present with bvFTD-type dementia
- Early cognitive decline
- Early frontal behavioral dysfunction
- Motor symptoms absent for first few years

PSP-C
- Present initially with cerebellar ataxia
- Axial rigidity
- Early eye movement abnormalities
- Early postural instability

PSP-PAGF
- Early gait disturbance (including start hesitation and subsequent freezing)
- Axial rigidity
- Difficulty initiating/completing speech/writing
- Tremor rigidity, dementia, and eye movement abnormalities rare during first 5 years

---

FIGURE 3.24. Due to the heterogeneity in severity and distribution of tau pathology and neuron loss, PSP may present with a few distinct clinical phenotypes including PSP-Richardson's syndrome (PSP-RS); PSP-parkinsonism (PSP-P); PSP—pure akinesia with gait freezing (PSP-PAGF); PSP-corticobasal syndrome (PSP-CBS); PSP-speech and language (PSP-SL); PSP-frontal presentation (PSP-F); and PSP-predominant cerebellar ataxia (PSP-C). PSP-RS tends to have the greatest severity in terms of both tau pathology and disease. Of the PSP subtypes, only PSP-P seems to have any response to levodopa therapy (albeit moderate and transient) (Boxer et al, 2017; Ling, 2016; Kobylecki et al, 2015; Deutschlander et al, 2018; Williams et al, 2007).

Clinical Differentiation of PSP

Compared to PD, patients with PSP may have:
More behavioral symptoms such as apathy and disinhibition
Limited or absent response to levodopa
Eventual progression of PSP-P symptoms to PSP-RS symptoms
Fewer visual hallucinations
Eye movement abnormalities such as vertical gaze palsy
Hummingbird and/or morning glory signs on MRI

FIGURE 3.25. As many patients with PSP exhibit parkinsonian features at the onset of the disease, differentiating PSP from Parkinson's disease (PD) can be somewhat challenging, especially early in the disease course. However, there are several clinical features that can aid in the differentiation of PSP from PD. Adding challenge to the differential diagnosis is the fact that PSP often overlaps with other disorders; in patients with PSP, 36% have comorbid AD, 20% have comorbid PD, 1% have comorbid DLB, 44% have comorbid argyrophilic grain disease (AGD), and 25% have cerebral amyloid angiopathy (CAA) (Boxer et al, 2017; Kobylecki et al, 2015; Liscic et al, 2013; Ling, 2016).

PSP-RS: Hummingbirds and Morning Glories

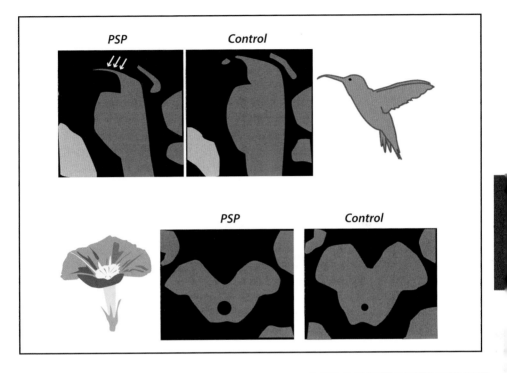

FIGURE 3.26. Two unique and classic findings on magnetic resonance images (MRI) in PSP (especially PSP-RS) are the "hummingbird sign" and the "morning glory sign." The hummingbird sign is due to greater midbrain atrophy relative to atrophy of the pons, while the morning glory sign is due to atrophy in the midbrain tegmentum; both of these atrophy patterns are common in PSP. Thus MRI can be very useful in differentiating PSP from other disorders (including Parkinson's disease, dementia with Lewy bodies, multiple system atrophy, and corticobasal degeneration) when clinical symptoms (e.g., parkinsonism, cognitive decline) overlap (Liscic et al, 2013; Meyer et al, 2017).

Corticobasal Degeneration

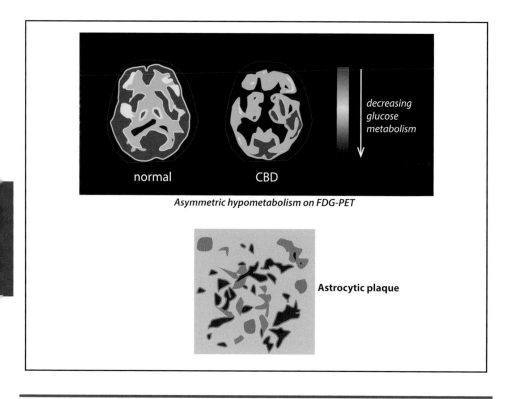

decreasing glucose metabolism

normal   CBD

Asymmetric hypometabolism on FDG-PET

Astrocytic plaque

FIGURE 3.27. Many patients with corticobasal degeneration (CBD) exhibit asymmetric atrophy in frontal and parietal cortices as well as basal ganglia, thalamus, and subthalamic nuclei. Clinically, patients with CBD present with corticobasal syndrome (with asymmetric parkinsonism, dystonia, apraxia, and alien limb phenomenon), bvFTD, nfvPPA, or some combination thereof. The phantom limb phenomenon, which usually occurs in one arm, is a classic sign of CBD; although the exact neurobiological substrate of this phantom limb phenomenon is not fully understood, it is hypothesized to result from combined damage to both motor and sensory cortices. Pathologically, there is accumulation of hyperphosphorylated 4R tau in both neurons and glia, which present histopathologically as ballooned neurons and astrocytic plaques (Dugger and Dickson, 2017; Mackenzie and Neumann, 2016; Tsai and Boxer, 2017; Buoli et al, 2017; Deutschlander and Wszolek, 2017; Eusebio et al, 2016).

Argyrophilic Grain Disease

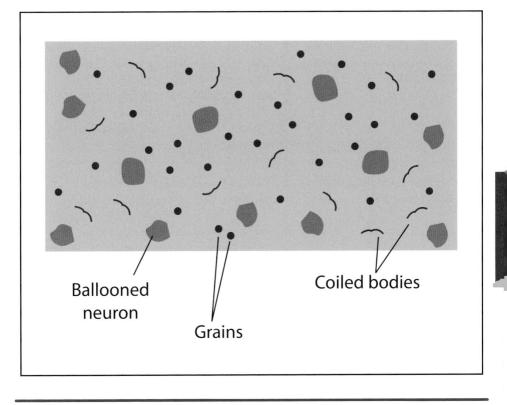

Ballooned neuron

Grains

Coiled bodies

FIGURE 3.28. Argyrophilic grain disease (AGD) often co-occurs with other FTLD-Tau disorders such as PSP and CBD and may be present in as many as 50% of individuals over the age of 80 years. It is a type of sporadic tauopathy that presents clinically with late-onset, slowly progressive, mild amnesic dementia with personality and emotional changes. Pathologically, patients with AGD exhibit spindle-shaped, argyrophilic 4R tau inclusions (termed "grains") in neuronal processes (hypothesized to represent degenerating dendrites) along with coiled bodies in glial cells and ballooned neurons most notably in the amygdala and temporal entorhinal cortex (Dugger and Dickson, 2017; Mackenzie and Neumann, 2016; Deutschlander et al, 2018; Togo et al, 2005).

FTLD Rating Scales

Frontotemporal Lobar Degeneration-Specific Version of the Clinical Dementia Rating (FTLD-CDR)	In addition to assessing the original 6 domains of cognitive and functional performance in the CRD (including memory, orientation, judgment and problem solving, community affairs, home and hobbies, and personal care), the FTLD-CDR assesses 2 additional domains: language and behavior, and comportment and personality
Frontotemporal Dementia Rating Scale (FRS)	This 30-item scale assesses 7 functional domains including behavior, outing and shopping, household chores and telephone, finances, medications, meal preparation and eating, and self-care and mobility
Frontal Behavior Inventory (FBI)	This 24-item scale is a behavioral inventory assessing deficit behaviors (apathy, aspontaneity, indifference, inflexibility, concreteness, personal neglect, disorganization, inattention, loss of insight, logopenia, verbal apraxia, and alien hand) as well as disinhibition behaviors (perseveration, excessive/childish jocularity, irresponsibility, inappropriateness, impulsivity, restlessness, aggression, hyperorality, hypersexuality, utilization behavior, and incontinence)

FIGURE 3.29. Several clinical rating scales have been developed to aid in the differential diagnosis and measurement of disease progression of FTLD disorders. These include the FTLD-Specific Version of the Clinical Dementia Rating Scale, the Frontotemporal Dementia Rating Scale, and the Frontal Behavior Inventory (Mioshi et al, 2017; Mioshi et al, 2010; Knopman et al, 2008; Kertesz and Munoz, 2002).

FTLD Treatment

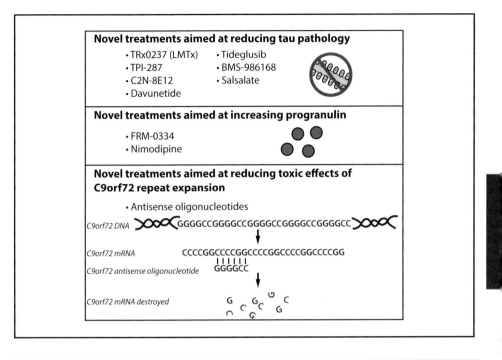

FIGURE 3.30. As with AD and LBDs, there are currently no disease-modifying agents available for any of the FTLD disorders, and treatments at this point are purely symptomatic (see Chapter 5). In addition to the novel tau-modifying strategies for AD (discussed in Chapter 5) and potential applicability for FTLD-Tau disorders, additional avenues of research include increasing progranulin levels in individuals with GRN mutations and using antisense oligonucleotides in patients with pathological C9orf72 repeat expansions. Unfortunately, the cholinesterase inhibitors and memantine that are used to stabilize cognitive decline AD, and even LBDs, are not recommended for patients with FTLDs as they are ineffective and may actually worsen behavioral symptoms, cognition, and motor function. Physical therapy, exercise, and dopamine replacement therapy may provide some relief (albeit limited) for patients with FTLDs and motor symptoms (Tsai and Boxer, 2016; Buoli et al, 2017).

| Chapter 4

Other Dementias

In Chapter 4, we discuss the various types of dementia that do not readily fall into the Alzheimer's, Lewy body dementias, or frontotemporal lobar degeneration disorders discussed in Chapters 1–3. In addition to reviewing some of the causes of dementia that may be reversible in nature, Chapter 4 also covers vascular dementia, prion disease, chronic traumatic encephalopathy, dementia related to HIV infection, and dementia associated with Huntington's disease. For strategies to ameliorate some of the secondary behavioral symptoms often associated with all types of dementia, the reader is directed to Chapter 5.

Vascular Dementia

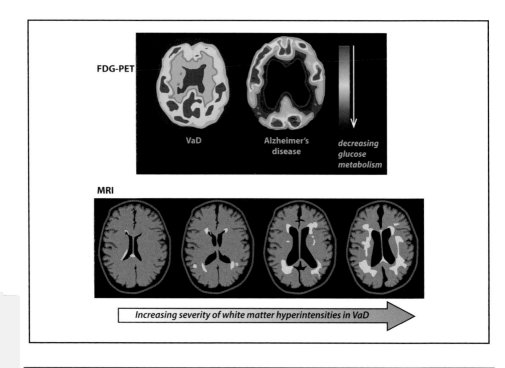

FIGURE 4.1. Vascular dementia (VaD), the 2nd most common form of dementia, accounts for 20% of dementia cases and is essentially a neurological manifestation of cardiovascular disease. In VaD there is a decrease in cerebral blood flow, attributable to myriad pathologies including atherosclerosis, arteriosclerosis, infarcts, white matter changes, and microbleeds as well as deposition of amyloid beta protein into cerebral blood vessels (i.e., cerebral amyloid angiopathy or CAA). Many of the risk factors associated with peripheral cardiovascular disease (e.g., hypertension, smoking, heart disease, high cholesterol) are also linked with VaD. In fact, approximately 30% of elderly individuals who have a stroke will experience post-stroke cognitive impairment and/or dementia. There is often significant overlap between VaD and AD; however, "pure VaD" cases show a different pattern of hypoperfusion on FDG-PET with hypometabolism in the sensorimotor and subcortical areas and a relative sparing of the association cortex (Allan et al, 2017; Chutinet and Rost, 2014; Yang et al, 2017; Maloney and Lahiri, 2016; Jena et al, 2015).

Cerebral Amyloid Angiopathy (CAA)

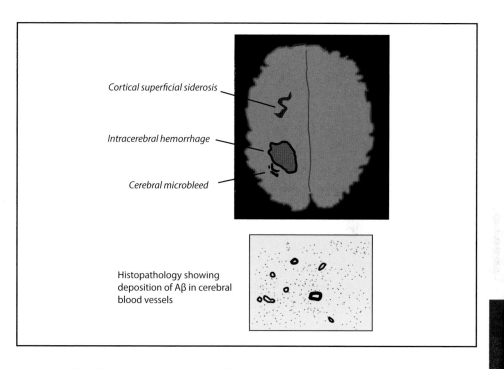

Cortical superficial siderosis

Intracerebral hemorrhage

Cerebral microbleed

Histopathology showing deposition of Aβ in cerebral blood vessels

FIGURE 4.2. Cerebral amyloid angiopathy (CAA) is a type of VaD in which amyloid β protein (particularly Aβ40) is deposited into blood vessel walls within the brain. This Aβ accumulation leads to disruption of the blood–brain barrier. As many as 90% of patients with Alzheimer's disease (AD) have comorbid CAA; however, CAA (and the cognitive dysfunction it can cause) can occur in the absence of AD. Similar to AD, risk for CAA is affected by apolipoprotein E (APOE) genotype, with the APOEε4 allele increasing risk and the APOEε2 allele conveying the greatest risk of CAA (Kovari et al, 2013; Greenberg and Charidimou, 2018; DeSimone et al, 2017).

Diagnosing CAA

Modified Boston Criteria for the Diagnosis of CAA

PROBABLE CAA WITH SUPPORTING PATHOLOGY

Clinical data and pathological tissue demonstrating:
- Lobar, cortical, or cortical–subcortical hemorrhage
  - Cortical superficial siderosis (cSS)
  - Intracerebral hemorrhage (ICH)
  - Cerebral microbleed (CMB)
- Some degree of CAA in specimen
- Absence of other diagnostic lesion

PROBABLE CAA

Clinical data and MRI or CT showing:
- Multiple hemorrhages restricted to lobar, cortical, or cortical–subcortical regions or single lobar, cortical, or cortical–subcortical hemorrhage and cSS
- Age ≥55 years
- Absence of other cause of hemorrhage

POSSIBLE CAA

Clinical data and MRI or CT showing:
- Single lobar, cortical, or cortical–subcortical ICH, CMB, or cSS
- Age ≥55 years
- Absence of other cause of hemorrhage

FIGURE 4.3. Although CAA can only be definitely diagnosed with postmortem analysis, the Modified Boston Criteria for the diagnosis of CAA provide guidelines for making diagnoses of possible or probable CAA with increasing level of certainty based on clinical presentation, histopathology in a biopsy specimen, and magnetic resonance and computed tomography (MRI/CT) neuroimaging (Kovari et al, 2013; Greenberg and Charidimou, 2018; DeSimone et al, 2017).

AD/VaD Comorbidity

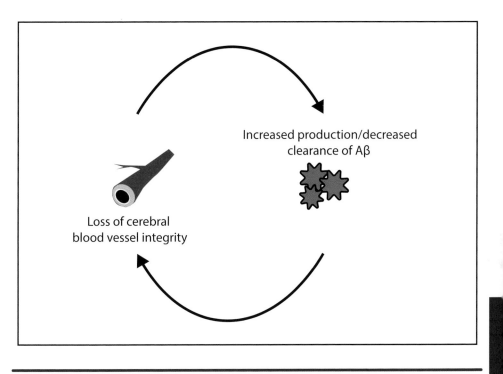

Increased production/decreased clearance of Aβ

Loss of cerebral blood vessel integrity

FIGURE 4.4. A large portion of individuals with Alzheimer's disease have comorbid VaD pathology, and this overlap is hypothesized to occur due to a dynamic relationship between amyloid metabolism and cerebral vasculature integrity. According to this hypothesis, the deposition of amyloid beta into cerebral blood vessels increases risk for VaD; conversely, loss of integrity and increased permeability of the blood–brain barrier has been shown to increase production and reduce clearance of amyloid beta (Chakraborty et al, 2017; Raz et al, 2016; Schott et al, 2011).

Creutzfeldt–Jakob Disease (CJD)

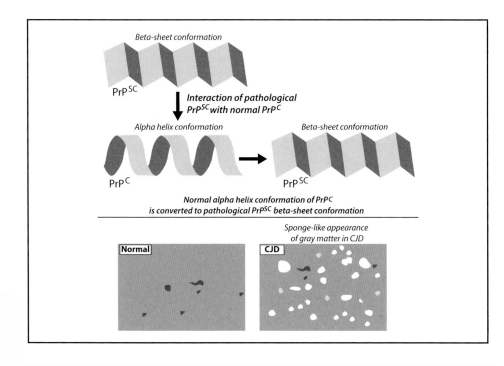

FIGURE 4.5. Creutzfeldt–Jakob disease (CJD) is a type of proteinaceous infectious particle (a.k.a., prion) disease that causes a rapidly progressing dementia with memory loss, executive dysfunction, and language impairments, as well as parkinsonism and behavioral symptoms. The pathology of CJD involves misfolded PrPSC (SC standing for "scrapie") beta-sheet conformation proteins which are able to propagate by causing the misfolding of neighboring alpha-helix conformation PrPC (where C stands for "cellular") proteins. The brain of a patient with CJD has a spongy appearance due to neurodegeneration in cerebral, subcortical, and cerebellar gray matter and, like most other forms of dementia, CJD is irreversible. Interestingly, it has been suggested that diseases such as AD, PD, ALS, MSA, and Huntington's disease (HD), all of which involve misfolded proteins, may also spread through the brain in a prion-like manner (Annus et al, 2016; Burchell and Panegyres, 2016; Hasegawa et al, 2017; Hinz and Geschwind, 2017; Llorens et al, 2017; Takada et al, 2017).

Chronic Traumatic Encephalopathy

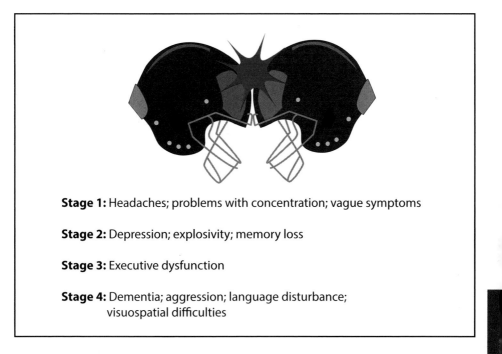

Stage 1: Headaches; problems with concentration; vague symptoms

Stage 2: Depression; explosivity; memory loss

Stage 3: Executive dysfunction

Stage 4: Dementia; aggression; language disturbance; visuospatial difficulties

FIGURE 4.6. Approximately 30% of individuals exposed to chronic, repetitive head trauma will develop chronic traumatic encephalopathy (CTE) (a.k.a., punch drunk syndrome or dementia pugilistica). Patients with CTE exhibit deficits in executive, visuospatial, memory, and/or language domains following head trauma; individuals with a lifetime history of head trauma have a 63% increased risk of developing any type of dementia, including Alzheimer's disease (AD). Unlike AD, CTE is conceptualized as a tauopathy with tau pathology, rather than Aβ pathology, predominant in the cortex and hippocampus, although Aβ pathology is often also present. Clinically, the presentation of CTE frequently begins with headaches and problems concentrating, progressing to depression, explosivity, memory loss, executive dysfunction, and, finally, dementia, aggression, and language disturbance (Arendt et al, 2016; Li et al, 2017; Asken et al, 2016; Dugger and Dickson, 2017; Motenigro et al, 2014).

Huntington's Disease (HD)

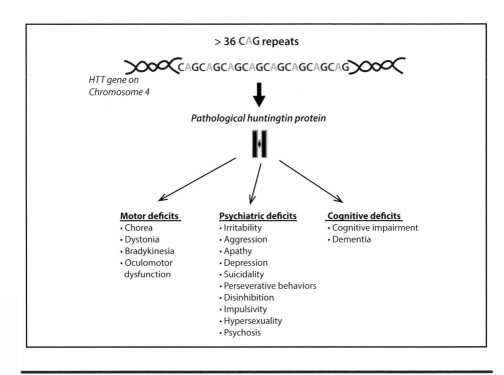

FIGURE 4.7. Huntington's disease (HD), also called Huntington's chorea, is a progressive neurodegenerative autosomal dominant disorder in which patients (typically age 35–45 years) present with severe motor, cognitive, and psychiatric deficits. Pathologically, HD is due to the build-up of aberrant huntingtin protein, although tau pathology may also be seen in as many as 60% of patients. Neuron loss in HD is largely located within the caudate nucleus and putamen, although cortical areas, thalamus, hypothalamus, and cerebellum are also commonly affected. Pathological huntingtin protein is made due to a CAG repeat expansion within the huntingtin (HTT) gene located on chromosome 4. As is typically the case in neurodegenerative diseases, there is currently no effective therapy for HD and treatment is purely symptomatic (Arendt et al, 2016; Eddy et al, 2016; Paoli et al, 2017; Tyebi and Hannan, 2017).

Reversible Dementia

Cause
Post-traumatic hydrocephalus
Drug or alcohol toxicity
Electrolyte imbalance
B12 deficiency
Intracranial bleeding
Thyroid disorders
HIV-related dementia

FIGURE 4.8. Although the vast majority of dementia cases have causes that are progressive and irreversible, there are some cases of dementia caused by factors that, when properly treated, can remit. It is important to rule out such reversible factors when making any differential diagnosis in a patient presenting with dementia or mild cognitive impairment, as these cases account for approximately 9% of all dementias (Alzheimer's Association, 2017; Allan et al, 2017; Pandya et al, 2016).

Delirium

PRESENTATION

- Confused/bizarre mental status
- Clouded sensorium and inattentiveness
- Confusion and disorientation
- Impaired short-term memory
- Visual/tactile hallucinations
- Occasional olfactory hallucinations
- Impaired judgment and social skills
- Variable degrees of paranoia
- Disturbed behavior

POTENTIAL CAUSES

Metabolic disorders
- Hypoxia
- Hypoglycemia
- Electrolyte imbalance
- Alcohol or sedative withdrawal
- Endocrine disorders
- Hyper- or hypothermia
- Post-operative anesthesia

Other
- Fever
- Postictal states
- Urinary retention
- Fecal impaction

Infections

Toxins
- Alcohol or illicit drugs
- Medications
- Anticholinergic toxicity
- Herbal supplements
- Poison

Anatomic disorders
- Brain lesion
- Tumor
- Trauma

Environmental disorders
- Sensory deprivation
- Sleep deprivation

FIGURE 4.9. As many as 13–89% of patients with dementia also present with delirium; however, delirium is not always present in patients with dementia and can be distinguished from dementia and possibly reversed (e.g., if due to electrolyte imbalance). While both dementia and delirium may present clinically with memory deficits, impaired judgment, confusion, disorientation, and psychosis, in delirium the presentation is usually acute and fluctuating and more often includes cloudiness of consciousness and sleep disturbances, most notably circadian rhythm disturbances. In most cases, the treatment of delirium involves addressing the underlying cause(s) (Lippmann and Perugula, 2016; Ford, 2016).

Alcohol-Related Dementia

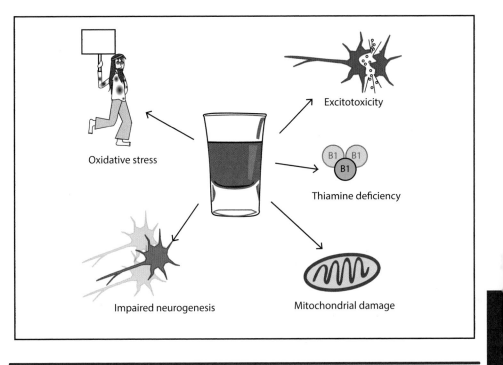

FIGURE 4.10. Although moderate alcohol consumption can actually lower one's risk of dementia, the excessive and prolonged use of alcohol can lead to alcohol-related dementia (ARD), which accounts for approximately 10% of all cases of dementia. The permanent damage to the brain caused by excessive alcohol consumption is hypothesized to be due to a number of factors including the direct neurotoxic effects of alcohol, oxidative stress, excitotoxicity, disruption of neurogenesis, compromised thiamine metabolism, and mitochondrial damage (Sachdeva et al, 2016; Venkataraman et al, 2017).

Wernicke–Korsakoff Syndrome (WKS)

Compared to AD, patients with WKS may have:
Fewer language impairments
Better confrontational naming
Better category fluency
Better semantic memory
Better verbal memory

Compared to healthy individuals, patients with WKS may have:
Poorer visuospatial skills
Poorer verbal abstract reasoning and letter fluency
Poorer working memory
Decreased motor speed
Antegrade amnesia
Impaired recall

FIGURE 4.11. Wernicke's encephalopathy (WE) is an acute form of alcohol-related dementia that often presents with ophthalmoplegia (paralysis of muscles surrounding the eye), ataxia (loss of body movement control), and confusion with neuron loss and lesions in the periventricular and periaqueductal gray matter. As WE progresses, it can turn into Korsakoff's syndrome (KS), which includes profound memory loss accompanied by damage to the diencephalic and hippocampal circuitry. Although many cases of Wernicke–Korsakoff syndrome (WKS) are permanent and progressive, prolonged abstinence from alcohol, administration of thiamine, memantine, and cognitive rehabilitation may reverse some of this alcohol-related dementia (Sachdeva et al, 2016; Venkataraman et al, 2017).

HIV-Associated Dementia

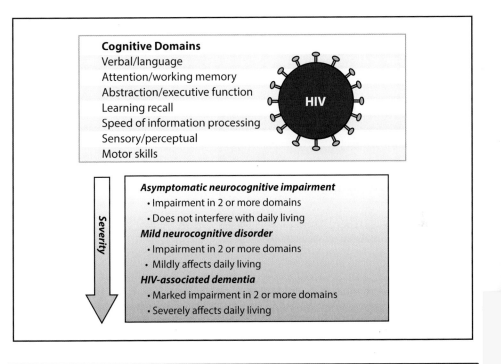

FIGURE 4.12. Human immunodeficiency virus (HIV) is classically thought of as being associated with an immunologic disorder; however, a large portion of patients infected with HIV also exhibit some cognitive dysfunction. It is hypothesized that neurocognitive deficits, which span from mild to dementia, are due to the presence of HIV in the brain and consequent chronic macrophage activation and neuronal injury. Fortunately, there has been a decline in cases of severe HIV-associated dementia, owing to the advent of effective antiretroviral treatments for HIV infection. While these treatments may not entirely reverse (or prevent) neurocognitive dysfunction, they do appear to allow patients to avoid the most severe manifestations of HIV-related cognitive impairment and dementia (Farhadian et al, 2017).

Normal Pressure Hydrocephalus

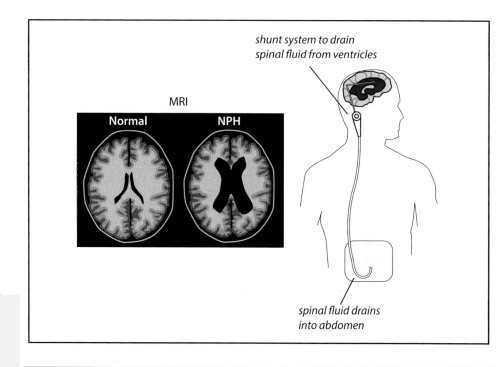

FIGURE 4.13. Normal pressure hydrocephalus (NPH), which accounts for less than 5% of dementia cases, is a condition in which cerebrospinal fluid (CSF) builds up within the ventricles of the brain, causing significant pressure throughout the brain. Although some cases of NPH are secondary and due to, e.g., traumatic brain injury or meningitis, most cases are idiopathic and believed to be caused by impaired resorption of CSF. Patients with NPH typically present with gait impairments, cognitive dysfunction, including memory loss, and urinary incontinence, which can be difficult to distinguish from other causes of dementia. Surgical placement of a shunt that drains CSF from the ventricles into the abdomen can sometimes reverse the symptoms of NPH, most notably gait disturbances; however, oftentimes dementia and urinary incontinence are irreversible (Deutschlander et al, 2018; McGirt et al, 2005).

Mixed Dementia

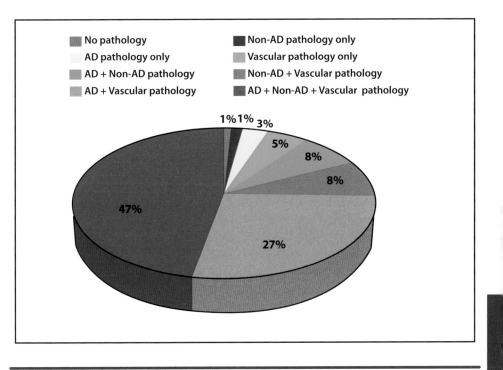

FIGURE 4.14. While we categorize dementias clinically based on their suspected etiologies, in fact, dementias with only one type of pathology are likely the exception rather than the rule. Even in cases diagnosed as probable AD, most postmortem pathological analyses reveal mixed pathology including both vascular pathology and non-AD pathology (including Lewy bodies and TDP-43 pathology). It is hypothesized that this mixed pathology lowers the threshold for cognitive impairment, either through additive or synergistic mechanisms, with each type of pathology potentially contributing to deficits in different (as well as overlapping) cognitive and behavioral domains (Alzheimer's Association; Kapasi et al, 2017).

Treatment of Secondary Behavioral Symptoms of Dementia

As we have seen, the majority of dementias have no disease-altering therapeutic interventions currently available. Treatment options are thus limited to symptomatic presentations and strive to relieve patients and caregivers of some of the behavioral and psychiatric sequelae that can severely impact the quality of life. In fact, neuropsychiatric symptoms of dementia affect virtually all patients with dementia at some time during the disease course and are associated with earlier institutionalization, increased caregiving costs (both financial and otherwise), and worsened disease progression. Unfortunately, pharmacological measures acting on neurocircuitry that may be damaged in the brains of patients with dementia as well as attempts to utilize non-pharmacological, cognition-acting strategies in cognitively impaired patients with dementia may not be as effective as they are for younger, non-demented patients. It is also important to note that improvements in behavioral symptoms (e.g., depression) may be due not solely to a prescribed psychotropic agent but may also be a result of the extra social contact with the treatment team that medication warrants.

In this chapter, we will discuss some of the behavioral symptoms of dementia as well as treatments that may be potentially therapeutic or potentially contraindicated. It should be noted that first-line treatment of any behavioral symptom associated with dementia should always be non-pharmacological. We will also address a very important issue—namely the well-being of those who care for patients living with dementia (Lanctot et al, 2017; Cepoiu-Martin et al, 2016; Hongisto et al, 2018; Van der Linde et al, 2016).

Assessing Neuropsychiatric Symptoms in Dementia

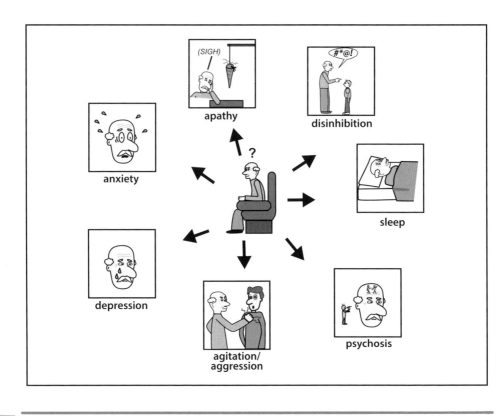

FIGURE 5.1. The Neuropsychiatric Inventory Questionnaire (NPI) is an excellent resource for evaluating not only the severity of a variety of secondary behavioral symptoms associated with dementia but also the impact that such behaviors have on the caregiver. For each behavior, severity is rated on a scale of 1–3 (with one being mild) and caregiver distress is rated on a scale of 0–5 (with zero being not distressing at all) (Lanctot et al, 2017; http://npitest.net/ Accessed March 1, 2018).

Non-pharmacological Options for Behavioral Symptoms in Dementia

- Address unmet needs (hunger, pain, thirst, boredom)
- Identify/modify environmental stressors
- Identify/modify daily routine stressors
- Caregiver support/training
- Behavior modification
- Group/individual therapy
- Problem solving
- Distraction
- Provide outlets for pent-up energy (exercise, activities)
- Avoid behavior triggers
- Increase social engagement
- Relaxation techniques
- Reminiscence therapy
- Music therapy
- Aromatherapy
- Pet therapy

FIGURE 5.2. There are several non-pharmacological options for treating neuropsychiatric symptoms in patients with dementia, and given the risks associated with many pharmacological treatments, non-pharmacological interventions should always be considered first-line (Goodarzi et al, 2016; Porteinsson and Antonsdottir, 2017; Lanctot et al, 2017; Macfarlane and O'Connor, 2016; Cheston and Ivanecka, 2017; Zhang et al, 2017).

Pain

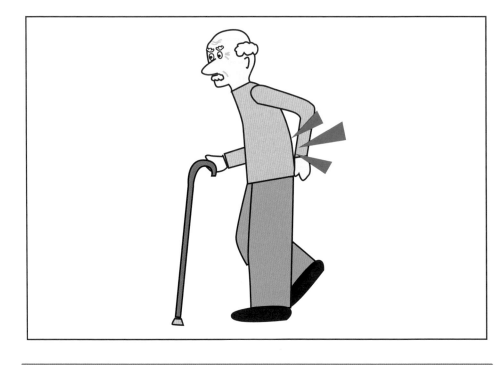

FIGURE 5.3. It is important to keep in mind that physical pain, infection, or local irritation can be the underlying cause for many secondary behavioral symptoms in patients with dementia. Just as with household pets or small children, a patient with dementia may not be able to express or describe the physical pain they are experiencing; thus it is up to astute clinicians and caregivers to identify and treat causes of pain that may be leading to neuropsychiatric symptoms, such as agitation and depression, in patients with dementia. If pain is contributing to behavioral symptoms, psychotropic medications may have little effect whereas alleviating the source of the pain may be quite effective. For instance, treatment with simple acetaminophen can sometimes ameliorate agitation. Similarly, other modifiable sources of behavioral symptoms (e.g., boredom, excess stimulation, etc.) should be recognized and addressed (Lochhead et al, 2016; Macfarlane and O'Connor, 2016; Ford and Almeida, 2017).

Rolling the DICE

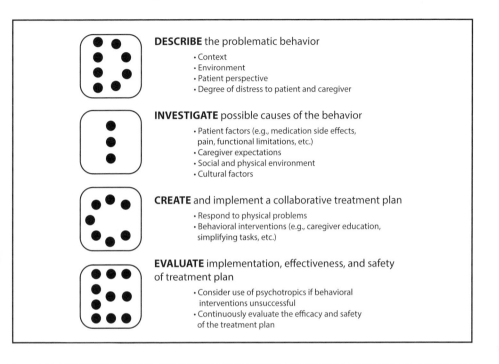

DESCRIBE the problematic behavior
- Context
- Environment
- Patient perspective
- Degree of distress to patient and caregiver

INVESTIGATE possible causes of the behavior
- Patient factors (e.g., medication side effects, pain, functional limitations, etc.)
- Caregiver expectations
- Social and physical environment
- Cultural factors

CREATE and implement a collaborative treatment plan
- Respond to physical problems
- Behavioral interventions (e.g., caregiver education, simplifying tasks, etc.)

EVALUATE implementation, effectiveness, and safety of treatment plan
- Consider use of psychotropics if behavioral interventions unsuccessful
- Continuously evaluate the efficacy and safety of the treatment plan

FIGURE 5.4. In approaching behavioral symptoms associated with dementia, the DICE plan (Describe, Investigate, Create, Evaluate) can be implemented. Note that this plan also recommends non-pharmacological interventions and seeks to find, and ameliorate, potentially modifiable causes (medical, environmental, etc.) of the behavior before initiating any psychotropic treatment (Fraker et al, 2014).

Hypothetical Associations between Depression and Dementia

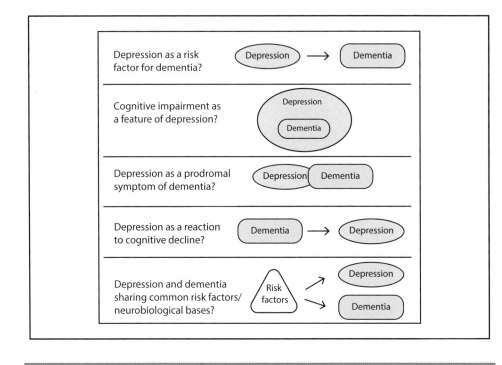

FIGURE 5.5. It is well-established that an association exists between depression and dementia; however, the exact nature of this intricate relationship is not fully understood. Individuals with major depressive disorder (MDD) often complain of memory problems (so-called pseudodementia), which can sometimes be reversed but also may be a prodromal symptom of, or risk factor for, inevitable dementia. In fact, a history of MDD is associated with a 2-fold increase in the risk for developing dementia, particularly vascular dementia whereas MDD with an onset in later life may signify a prodromal sign of Alzheimer's disease. Additionally, symptoms of MDD are seen in at least 50% of individuals diagnosed with dementia and should be addressed whenever feasible (Bennett and Thomas, 2014; Tsuno and Homma, 2009; Caraci et al, 2010; Evan and Weintraub, 2010; Geerlings et al, 2008; Rapp et al, 2006; Bao et al, 2008; Wuwongse et al, 2010).

Assessment of Depression in Patients with Dementia

Dementia Mood Assessment Scale (DMAS)

- Self-directed motor activity
- Sleep
- Appetite
- Psychomotor complaints
- Energy
- Irritability
- Physical agitation
- Anxiety
- Depressed appearance
- Awareness of emotional state
- Emotional responsiveness
- Sense of enjoyment
- Self-esteem
- Guilt feelings
- Hopelessness/helplessness
- Suicidal ideation
- Speech
- Diurnal mood variation
- Diurnal cognitive variations
- Paranoid symptoms
- Other psychotic symptoms
- Expressive communication skills
- Receptive cognitive capacity
- Cognitive insight

Cornell Scale for Depression in Dementia (CSDD)

- Mood *(anxiety, sadness, anhedonia, irritability)*
- Behavioral disturbance *(agitation, retardation, physical complaints, lack of interest)*
- Physical signs *(appetite loss, weight loss, lack of energy)*
- Cyclic functions *(mood, sleep, awakening)*
- Ideational disturbance *(suicide, self-esteem, pessimism, delusion)*

Cornell Scale for Depression in Dementia (CSDD)

- Are you basically satisfied with your life?
- Have you dropped many of your activities and interests?
- Do you feel that your life is empty?
- Do you often get bored?
- Are you in good spirits most of the time?
- Are you afraid that something bad is going to happen to you?
- Do you feel happy most of the time?
- Do you often feel helpless?
- Do you prefer to stay at home, rather than going out and doing new things?
- Do you feel you have more problems with memory than most?
- Do you think it is wonderful to be alive now?
- Do you feel pretty worthless the way you are now?
- Do you feel full of energy?
- Do you feel that your situation is hopeless?
- Do you think that most people are better off than you are?

FIGURE 5.6. The Dementia Mood Assessment Scale (DMAS), the Cornell Scale for Depression in Dementia (CSDD), and the Geriatric Depression Scale (GDS) are commonly used tools for evaluating depression in older patients with dementia. Both the DMAS and the CSDD can be administered by a caregiver or family member with regular interaction with the patient while the GDS can be completed by patients with mild-to-moderate dementia   (Alexopoulos et al, 1988; https://www.cambridge.org/core Accessed March 4, 2018; https://web.stanford.edu/~yesavage/GDS.html Accessed March 4, 2018; Goodarzi et al, 2016).

Treating Depression

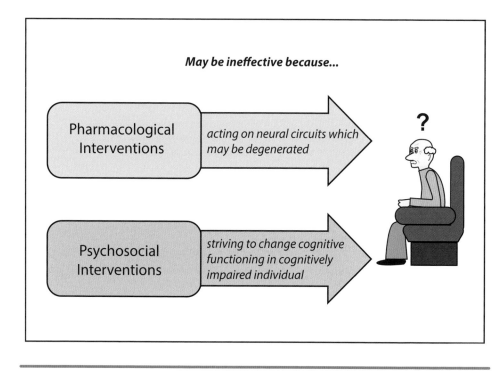

FIGURE 5.7. Given that symptoms of depression can significantly impact quality of life for patients with dementia and may actually exacerbate cognitive decline, addressing depressive symptoms using non-pharmacological and/or pharmacological means should be a priority. Unfortunately, the treatment of depression in elderly patients with dementia may be complicated by the potential depression-exacerbating effects of medications for somatic ailments common in the elderly population, as well as the potential interactions of such medications with standard antidepressants (Ford and Almeida, 2017; Kok and Reynolds, 2017; Caraci et al, 2010; Tariot and Aisen, 2009; Yeh and Tsai, 2008; Mossello et al, 2008).

Selective Serotonin Reuptake Inhibitors (SSRIs)

SSRI	Dose (mg/day)
Sertraline	50–200
Citalopram	20–40
Escitalopram	10–20
Fluoxetine	20–80
Paroxetine	20–50

FIGURE 5.8. In terms of pharmacological management of MDD in patients with dementia, selective serotonin reuptake inhibitors (SSRIs) including sertraline, citalopram, escitalopram, and fluoxetine, have shown some limited efficacy. Although, in general, long-term antidepressant treatment has been associated with a lower risk of dementia, improved cognition and a slower rate of decline in elderly patients with dementia, there are some data suggesting that chronic use of SSRIs may be associated with an increased risk of dementia. However, it is entirely possible that chronic SSRI use over the lifetime represents a high degree of lifetime depression (a risk factor for dementia), suggesting that SSRI use in and of itself does not put one at increased risk of developing dementia. Data are somewhat inconclusive in terms of their efficacy in treating MDD in dementia; however, SSRIs (citalopram in particular) may have some additional applicability towards ameliorating agitation and inappropriate behaviors in patients with dementia. Although considered relatively tolerable, SSRIs may be associated with increased falls and osteoporosis and may have interactions with other medications. Additionally, SSRIs may worsen some symptoms of Parkinson's disease such as restless leg syndrome, periodic limb movements, and REM sleep behavior disorders. Therefore, if a trial of a SSRI (or any other antidepressant medication) is deemed necessary, the lowest effective dose should be used and continuous monitoring should be exercised (Kok and Reynolds, 2017; Moraros et al, 2017; Kessing et al, 2009; Mossello et al, 2008; Farina et al, 2017; Lochhead et al, 2016; Torrisi et al, 2017; Preuss et al, 2016; Stahl, 2017b).

Tricyclic Antidepressants (TCAs)

TCA	Dose (mg/day)
Clomipramine	100–200
Amitriptyline	50–150
Desipramine	100–200
Imipramine	50–150

FIGURE 5.9. Tricyclic antidepressants (TCAs) such as clomipramine, amitriptyline, and desipramine have a greater risk of adverse effects compared to SSRIs, including anticholinergic effects that may worsen cognition in patients with dementia. TCAs may have limited efficacy in treating depression in patients with dementia; however, some data exist supporting their efficacy in other secondary behavioral symptoms of dementia such as inappropriate sexual behavior (Goodarzi et al, 2016; Torrisi et al, 2017; Preuss et al, 2016; Stahl 2017b).

Monoamine Oxidase Inhibitors (MAOIs)

MAOI	Dose (mg/day)
Selegiline	5–10
Phenelzine	45–75
Tranylcypromine	30

FIGURE 5.10. Monoamine oxidase inhibitors (MAOIs) such as selegiline, phenelzine, and tranylcypromine have shown some limited efficacy in treating depression in patients with dementia; however, one must carefully consider the risks of potential concomitant food and medication interactions that might lead to serotonin syndrome, a potentially fatal elevation in serotonin levels (Goodarzi et al, 2016; Stahl 2017b).

Lithium

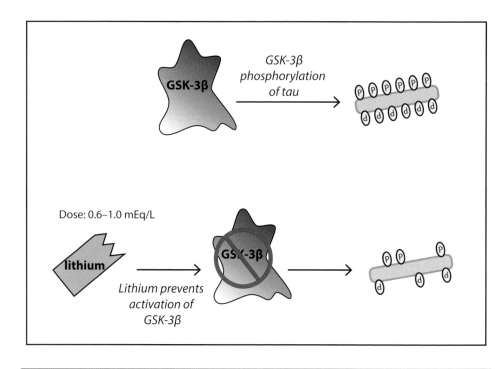

FIGURE 5.11. Lithium may be effective not only for depression in patients with dementia but may also hypothetically help with pathology in the dementias associated with tauopathy via its role in tau phosphorylation. Trials of lithium for symptoms of dementia have been inconclusive; however, some studies have suggested that the dose of lithium in trials for dementia was not high enough. Interestingly, trace levels of lithium in drinking water may be negatively correlated with both Alzheimer's disease and suicide rates. Aside from that, lithium should probably be initiated at lower doses (<0.6 mEq/L) for elderly patients, and one must be especially conscious of lithium toxicity (Bluml et al, 2013; Fajardo et al, 2018; Ford and Almeida, 2017; Tariot and Aisen, 2009; Yeh and Tsai, 2008; Stahl 2017b).

Anticonvulsants

Agent	Dose Range (mg/day)	Potential Side Effects
Valproate	500–1500	Sedation, tremor, dizziness, nausea, vomiting, diarrhea, reduced appetite, tachycardia, bradycardia, thrombocytopenia
Carbamazepine	400–1200	Sedation, dizziness, unsteadiness, confusion, nausea, vomiting
Lamotrigine	100–200	Rash, blurred vision, dizziness, sedation, headache, tremor, insomnia, nausea, vomiting

FIGURE 5.12. The anticonvulsants valproate, carbamazepine, and lamotrigine are often used to treat behavioral symptoms of dementia, particularly agitation, but have shown limited efficacy in ameliorating neuropsychiatric symptoms in patients with dementia. Additionally, these agents may be associated with significant side effects including sedation, unsteady gait, diarrhea, and weakness. Carbamazepine has perhaps shown the greatest efficacy in treating neuropsychiatric symptoms of dementia but has significant side effect risks and may interact with other medications commonly prescribed to elderly patients (Lochhead et al, 2016; Preuss et al, 2016; Torrisi et al, 2017; Stahl, 2017b).

Trazodone

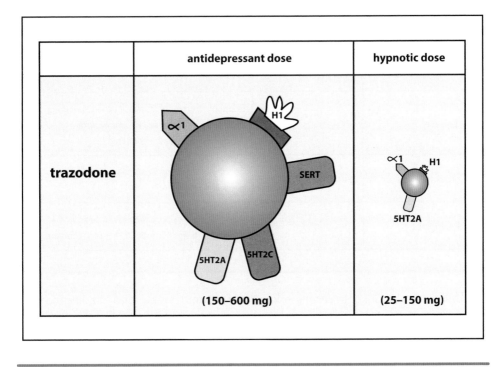

FIGURE 5.13. At antidepressant doses (150–600 mg/day), trazodone is a serotonin reuptake inhibitor and has serotonin 2A and 2C antagonism. In addition, trazodone is an antagonist at histamine H1 and alpha 1 adrenergic receptors, which can make it very sedating, particularly when given at antidepressant doses during the day. At low doses (25–150 mg/day), trazodone does not adequately block serotonin reuptake but retains its other properties; thus, it can still be sedating. However, because trazodone has a relatively short half-life (6–8 hours), if dosed only once daily at night, it can improve sleep without having daytime effects. The utility of trazodone in treating secondary behavioral symptoms in patients with dementia may lie more in its ability to improve sleep rather than depression (Stahl, 2013).

Cholinesterase Inhibitors and Memantine

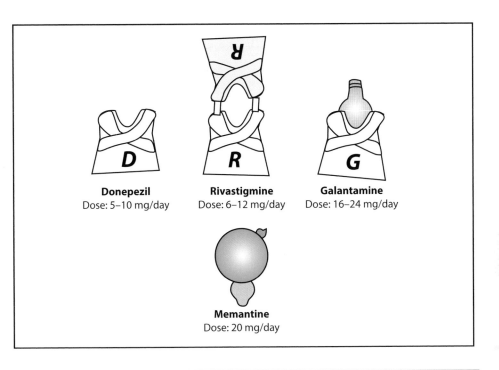

Donepezil
Dose: 5–10 mg/day

Rivastigmine
Dose: 6–12 mg/day

Galantamine
Dose: 16–24 mg/day

Memantine
Dose: 20 mg/day

FIGURE 5.14. While existing data do not support the use of cholinesterase inhibitors (ChEIs) or the NMDA antagonist memantine for depression in patients with dementia, many patients with dementia are nonetheless on these medications for cognitive decline. There is a glutamatergic hypothesis of depression in which aberrant glutamatergic neurotransmission is a pathological substrate for depressive symptoms; memantine, as a glutamatergic modulator, may help to alleviate symptoms of depression through its actions on the glutamatergic system (Ford and Almeida, 2017; Wuwongse et al, 2010; Stahl, 2017b; Gray and Hanlon, 2016).

Apathy

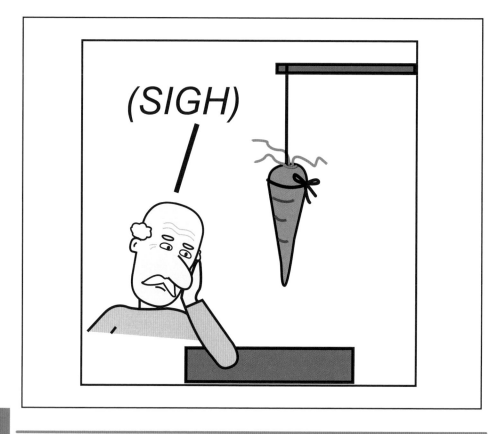

FIGURE 5.15. Apathy, characterized as diminished motivation and reduced goal-directed behavior, accompanied by decreased emotional responsiveness, affects approximately 90% of patients with dementia across the disease course. Apathy is indeed one of the most persistent and frequent secondary behavioral symptoms of dementia and has been shown to predict disease worsening and add tremendously to caregiver burden (Corcoran et al, 2004; Ducharme et al, 2018; Lyketsos et al, 2011; Marin et al, 1995).

Assessing Apathy

Lille Apathy Rating Scale
Reduction in everyday activity
Lack of interest
Lack of initiative
Extinction of novelty seeking
Motivation
Blunting of emotional responses
Lack of concern
Poor social life
Extinction of self-awareness

FIGURE 5.16. The Lille Apathy Rating Scale (LARS) consists of 33 items that are grouped into nine domains and can be used to assess characteristics of apathy including intellectual curiosity, emotion, action initiation, and self-awareness; the LARS has been validated for use in patients with dementia (Fernandez-Matarrubia et al, 2016).

Hypothesized Neurocircuitry and Treatment of Apathy

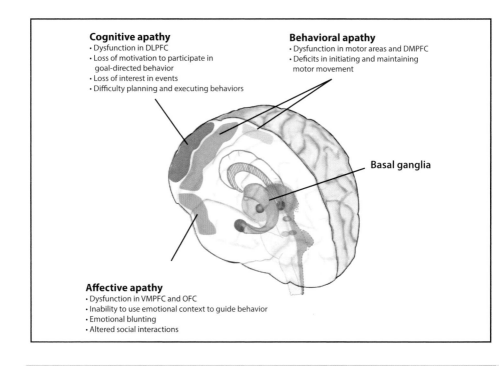

Cognitive apathy
• Dysfunction in DLPFC
• Loss of motivation to participate in goal-directed behavior
• Loss of interest in events
• Difficulty planning and executing behaviors

Behavioral apathy
• Dysfunction in motor areas and DMPFC
• Deficits in initiating and maintaining motor movement

Basal ganglia

Affective apathy
• Dysfunction in VMPFC and OFC
• Inability to use emotional context to guide behavior
• Emotional blunting
• Altered social interactions

FIGURE 5.17. The ABC (Affective/emotional, Behavioral, Cognitive) model of apathy categorizes 3 types of apathy, which can hypothetically be linked to deficits in different brain regions, as well as their connections to reward centers in the basal ganglia. The clinical presentation of apathy often differs among various types of dementias; for instance, affective apathy is more common in bvFTD compared to AD. Both dopaminergic and cholinergic neurotransmitter systems seem to be involved in the various types of apathy; potential treatments, therefore, include dopamine agonists such as bupropion, L-dopa, stimulants as well as cholinesterase inhibitors (Corcoran et al, 2004; Ducharme et al, 2018; Fernandez Kumfor et al, 2018; Matarrubia et al, 2018; Marin et al, 1995).

DLPFC: dorsolateral prefrontal cortex; DMPFC: dorsomedial prefrontal cortex; OFC: orbitofrontal cortex; VMPFC: ventromedial prefrontal cortex

Prevalence of Psychosis in Dementia

Prevalence of Psychosis	
Alzheimer's disease	25–40%
Dementia with Lewy bodies	75%
Parkinson's disease dementia	50–60%
Frontotemporal dementia	5–10%
Vascular dementia	15%

FIGURE 5.18. Symptoms of psychosis, including hallucinations and delusions, affect many individuals with varying types of dementia, especially in later stages of disease course. Although psychotic symptoms are often episodic and may resolve during the course of dementia, they can be quite troubling for caregivers and may increase the chance of institutionalization (Ballard et al, 2000; Ballard et al, 1995; Burns et al, 1990; Farina et al, 2017; Johnson et al, 2011; Lanctot et al, 2017; Lyketsos et al, 2002; Lyketsos et al, 2000; Leroi et al, 2003; Lopez et al, 2003; Preuss et al, 2016; Van der Linde et al, 2016).

Psychosis in AD vs. LBD

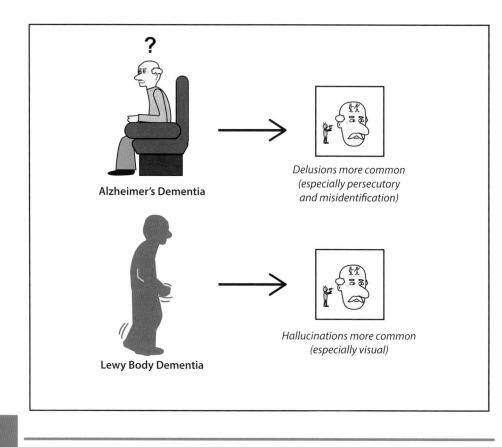

FIGURE 5.19. In Alzheimer's disease, delusions are more common than hallucinations whereas, in dementia with Lewy bodies, hallucinations are more common. Psychotic symptoms seem to be related to pathology in the neocortex, and specific symptoms (e.g., visual vs. auditory hallucinations) likely reflect damage to specific cortical areas (Farina et al, 2017; Lanctot et al, 2017; Preuss et al, 2016; Van der Linde et al, 2016).

Psychosis in Parkinson's Disease

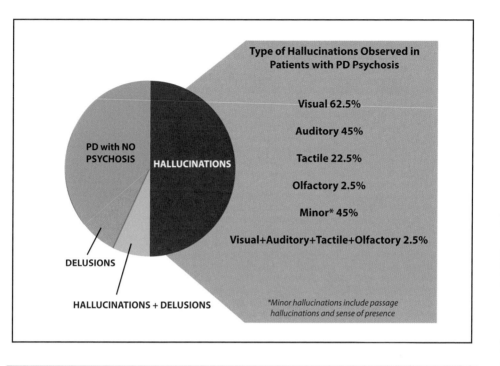

FIGURE 5.20. Psychosis is commonly associated with Parkinson's disease dementia (PDD) and is, in fact, one of the associated behavioral criteria indicative of probable PDD. The presence of psychosis often heralds the emergence of dementia (and vice versa) in patients with Parkinson's disease (PD), and up to 70% of patients with PDD report hallucinations (compared to only 10% of patients with PD but no dementia). Approximately 85% of patients with PD psychosis experience hallucinations only; 7.5% report both hallucinations and delusions; and 7.5% report delusions alone. The hallucinations reported by patients with PD are most often visual; however, other types of hallucinations may also be experienced (Amar et al, 2014; Anang et al, 2014; Goldman and Holden, 2014).

Neurobiological Basis of Psychosis: 3 Theories

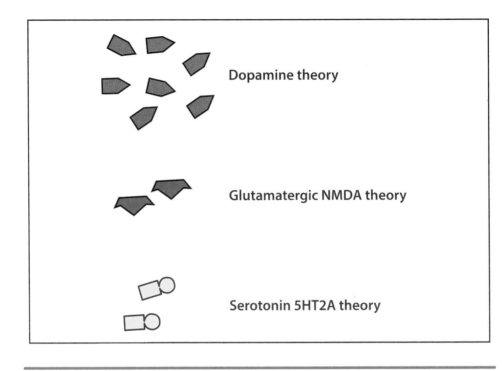

Dopamine theory

Glutamatergic NMDA theory

Serotonin 5HT2A theory

FIGURE 5.21. Psychosis is hypothesized to result from hyperactive dopamine D2 in the mesolimbic pathway, hypoactive serotonin 5HT2A in the cortex, and/or hypoactive glutamatergic NMDA receptors in the cortex. It is entirely possible that more than one of these dysfunctional circuits are the cause of psychosis in patients with dementia, especially as the underlying dementia-related pathology progresses and more brain areas become involved (Hacksell et al, 2014; Stahl, 2016).

Neurobiological Basis of Psychosis: Dopamine Theory

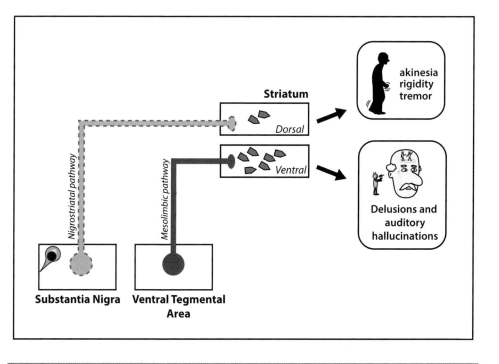

FIGURE 5.22. According to the dopamine D2 hypothesis of psychosis, dopaminergic projections along the mesolimbic pathway (dark blue; from the ventral tegmental area [VTA] to the ventral striatum) are hyperactive, leading to excess dopaminergic neurotransmission in the ventral striatum and resulting in psychosis, particularly delusions and auditory hallucinations. On the other hand, as neuropathology such as Lewy bodies leads to death of dopaminergic neurons of the nigrostriatal pathway (light blue; from the substantia nigra to the dorsal striatum), there is a paucity of dopaminergic input to the dorsal striatum, resulting in movement symptoms (Hacksell et al, 2014; Stahl, 2016).

Neurobiological Basis of Psychosis:
L-dopa, Dopamine, and Psychosis

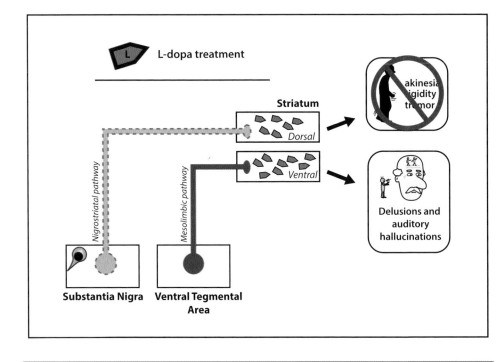

FIGURE 5.23. Dopamine replacement therapies, such as L-dopa, are often used to treat Parkinson's disease and reduce motor symptoms by increasing dopaminergic input in the dorsal striatum. However, L-dopa may also increase dopaminergic neurotransmission in the ventral striatum, leading to medication-associated psychotic symptoms (Hacksell et al, 2014; Stahl, 2016).

Neurobiological Basis of Psychosis: Antipsychotic Treatment

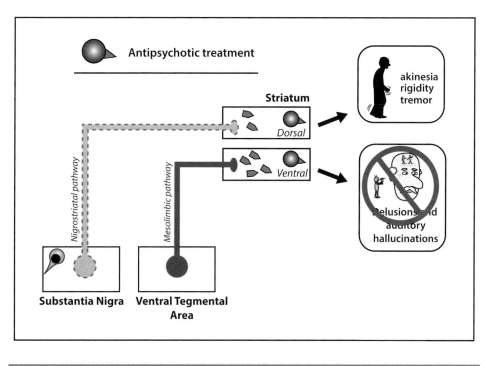

FIGURE 5.24. Treatment with a dopamine D2 receptor antagonist such as an antipsychotic can act in the ventral striatum to reduce dopaminergic input, thereby ameliorating symptoms of psychosis. However, the antipsychotic blockade of dopamine D2 receptors in the dorsal striatum may actually further reduce the already limited dopaminergic input from the substantia nigra, leading to worsening of motor symptoms (Hacksell et al, 2014; Stahl, 2016).

Neurobiological Basis of Psychosis: Glutamatergic NMDA Theory

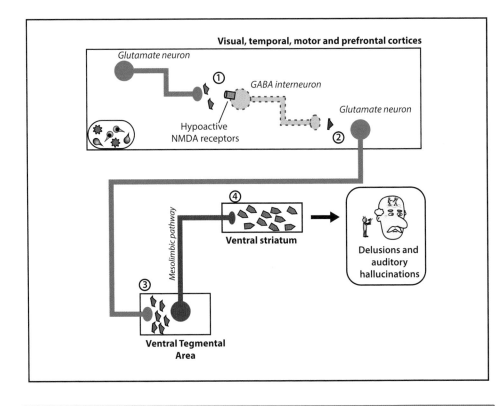

FIGURE 5.25. According to the glutamatergic NMDA hypothesis of psychosis, within the cerebral cortices (where amyloid, tau, or Lewy body neuropathology may be prevalent), (1) glutamatergic input to GABA interneurons is reduced due to hypoactive NMDA receptors located on GABA neurons. These GABA neurons are therefore not activated, leading to (2) reduced GABAergic input on downstream glutamatergic neurons (i.e., disinhibition. (3) Glutamatergic input onto, and thus activation of, dopaminergic neurons in the VTA occurs, leading to (4) excessive dopaminergic input to the ventral striatum and psychosis (Stahl, 2016).

Neurobiological Basis of Psychosis: Serotonin 5HT2A Theory

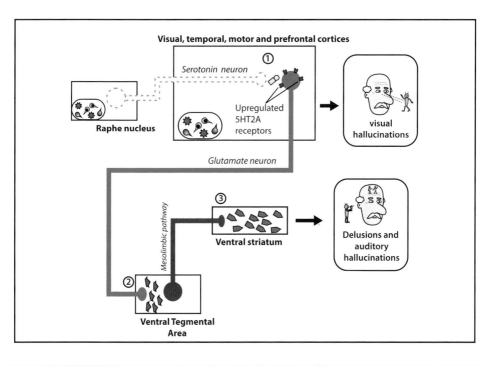

FIGURE 5.26. The serotonin 5HT2A hypothesis of psychosis posits that loss of serotonergic neurons in the raphe nuclei (due to Lewy body, amyloid, and/or tau pathology) leads to (1) hypoactive serotonergic neurotransmission in the cerebral cortices, which hypothetically causes upregulation of serotonin 5HT2A receptors located on glutamatergic neurons. This excessive glutamate, particularly in visual cortices, is thought to be the neurobiological substrate for visual hallucinations as are often seen in Parkinson's disease psychosis. (2) Glutamatergic input onto, and thus activation of, dopaminergic neurons in the VTA also occur, leading to (3) excessive dopaminergic input to the ventral striatum and psychosis (Stahl, 2016).

Treating Psychosis: Antipsychotics

Dosing Recommendations for Antipsychotics	
Haloperidol	6–40 mg/day
Risperidone	2–8 mg/day
Olanzapine	10–30 mg/day
Quetiapine	300–750 mg/day
Aripiprazole	10–30 mg/day
Clozapine	350 ng/mL trough plasma level

FIGURE 5.27. Conventional, first-generation antipsychotics (such as haloperidol) and the atypical, second-generation antipsychotics risperidone, olanzapine, quetiapine, and aripiprazole (all of which block dopamine D2 receptors) are commonly used to treat psychosis (and agitation) in patients with dementia. However, these agents may have limited efficacy and come with a wealth of side effect risks including weight gain and other cardiometabolic issues, anticholinergic-associated worsening of cognition, and sedation. Antipsychotics can also induce or worsen movement disorders via antagonism at dopamine D2 receptors in the dorsal striatum—which may worsen motor symptoms in patients with Parkinson's disease and other dementia types in which motor symptoms prevail. Importantly, the use of antipsychotics in elderly patients with dementia has been associated with an increased risk of mortality, warranting an FDA black box warning against their use in this population. For these reasons, it is recommended that antipsychotics only be used in cases where psychotic behavior is severe, potentially dangerous, and at the lowest dose possible for the smallest duration feasible (Lanctot et al, 2017; Lochhead et al, 2016; Preuss et al, 2016; Stahl 2017b; Stahl et al, 2014; Dennis et al, 2017).

Treating Psychosis: Pimavanserin

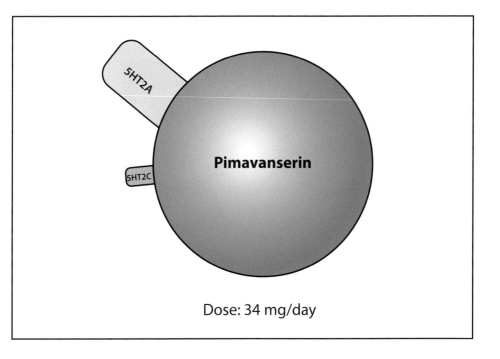

Dose: 34 mg/day

FIGURE 5.28. Pimavanserin, a novel serotonin 5HT2A and 5HT2C antagonist with no dopamine D2 binding affinity, is now approved for the treatment of psychosis in PD and appears to be effective in reducing visual hallucinations, without exacerbating motor effects. Side effects may include peripheral edema, confusion, nausea, and potential QTc prolongation. It remains to be seen whether pimavanserin has efficacy in treating psychosis associated with other forms of dementia such as Alzheimer's disease or all-cause dementia (Stahl, 2016b; Stahl 2017b).

Agitation

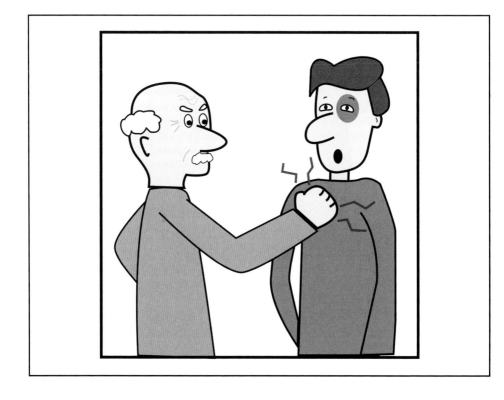

FIGURE 5.29. Agitation (encompassing emotional stress, excessive psychomotor activity, aggression, irritability, and disinhibition) is quite common in patients with dementia, affecting 50% or more of patients with Alzheimer's disease. First-line treatment involves addressing potential unmet needs that may be causing agitation, such as pain, hunger, or thirst (Porsteinsson and Antonsdottir, 2017; Lanctot et al, 2017; Farina et al, 2017; Garay and Grossberg, 2017; Lochhead et al, 2016; Torrisi et al, 2017).

Assessing Agitation

Cohen-Mansfield Agitation Inventory (CMAI)	
Physical/Aggressive	**Physical/Non-Aggressive**
Hitting	Pacing, aimless wandering
Kicking	Inappropriate dress/disrobing
Grabbing	Trying to get to a different place
Pushing	Intentional falling
Throwing things	Eating/drinking inappropriate substances
Biting	Handling things inappropriately
Scratching	Hiding things
Spitting	Hoarding things
Hurting self or others	Performing repetitive mannerisms
Destroying property	General restlessness
Making physical sexual advances	
Verbal/Aggressive	**Verbal/Non-Aggressive**
Screaming	Repetitive sentences or questions
Making verbal sexual advances	Strange noises
Cursing or verbal aggression	Complaining
	Negativism
	Constant unwarranted request for attention

FIGURE 5.30. Agitation can be conceptualized as physical and verbal behaviors that are excessive, inappropriate, repetitive, non-specific, and observable. The Cohen-Mansfield Agitation Inventory is a 29-item, clinician-rated, 7-point scale that can be used to assess both aggressive and non-aggressive verbal and physical behaviors indicating agitation (Cohen-Mansfield and Billig, 1986; Kong, 2005).

Hypothesized Neurobiology of Agitation and Aggression

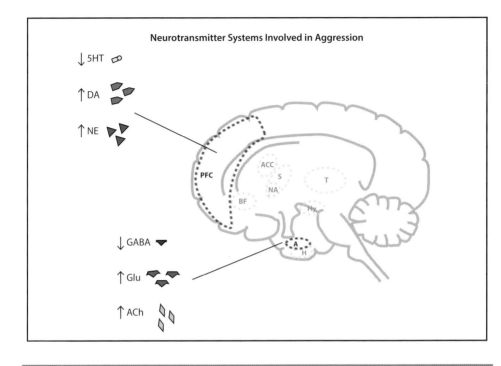

FIGURE 5.31. Agitation in patients with dementia may hypothetically stem from either impaired top-down cortical control of impulsive behaviors, irregular bottom-up drive from limbic regions, or as a result of psychosis. The neurotransmitters dopamine (DA), norepinephrine (NE), serotonin (5HT), acetylcholine (ACh), glutamate (Glu), and gamma-aminobutyric acid (GABA) are all thought to be involved in aggressive or agitated behaviors. In the prefrontal cortex (PFC) of aggressive/agitated patients, 5HT is hypothetically decreased, whereas both DA and NE are increased. In the limbic areas such as the amygdala (A) of aggressive/agitated patients, Glu and ACh are hypothetically increased whereas GABA is decreased. Pharmacological treatments for agitated behaviors thus seek to act on these aberrant neurotransmitter systems (Siever, 2008; Stahl and Morrissette, 2014).

Treating Agitation/Aggression

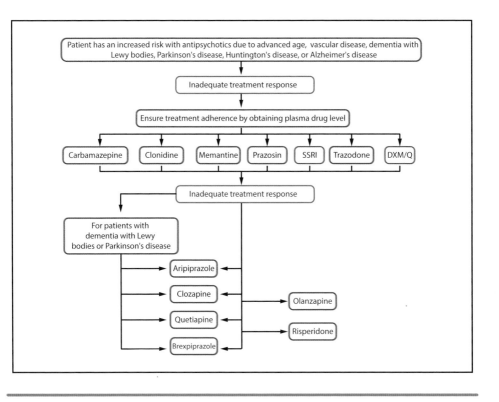

FIGURE 5.32. According to published expert consensus guidelines for the pharmacological treatment of violence in association with cognitive impairment, treatment of agitation and aggression in patients with dementia first involves non-antipsychotic-based therapies, with next-line measures including antipsychotic treatment. Note the importance of avoiding antipsychotics with a greater propensity for motor side effects in patients with Parkinson's disease dementia or other dementia types in which movement symptoms prevail (Stahl et al, 2014; Stahl and Morrissette, 2014; Preuss et al, 2016).

DXM/Q: dextromethorphan/quinidine

Dextromethorphan for Agitation/Aggression

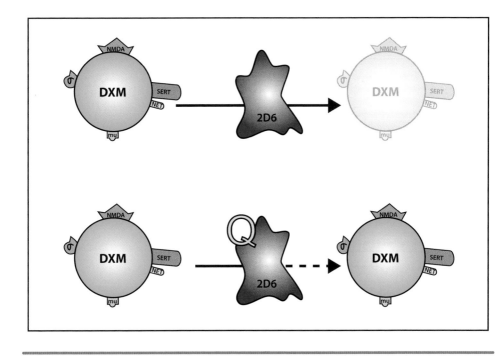

FIGURE 5.33. Dextromethorphan (DXM) is a sigma-1 and mu opiate receptor agonist with antagonist properties at NMDA and nicotinic α3β4 receptors and inhibition of both serotonin and norepinephrine reuptake inhibitors (SERT and NET, respectively). Dextromethorphan combined with quinidine (Q), which inhibits the cytochrome P450 2D6 (CYP 2D6) enzyme that metabolizes DXM, thereby increasing the bioavailability of DXM 20-fold, is FDA-approved for the treatment of pseudobulbar affect. Recent data have indicated that both dextromethorphan-quinidine and AVP-786, a deuterated version of DXM combined with a low dose of quinidine, may significantly reduce agitation in patients with Alzheimer's disease with relatively good tolerability. Deuteration of dextromethorphan reduces first-pass liver metabolism, slowing the rate of metabolism of dextromethorphan and allowing for an even lower dose of quinidine. The combination of dextromethorphan with the antidepressant bupropion, a norepinephrine and dopamine reuptake inhibitor and nicotinic acetylcholine receptor antagonist that has CYP 2D6-blocking capabilities and thus inhibits metabolism of dextromethorphan, is also being considered for treatment-resistant depression (Cummings et al, 2015; Garay and Grossberg, 2017).

Brexpiprazole for Agitation/Aggression

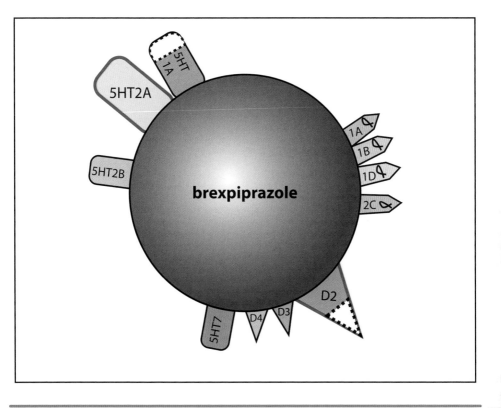

FIGURE 5.34. As a dopamine D2 receptor partial agonist, with dopamine D3, serotonin 5HT1A, serotonin 5HT2A, and adrenergic alpha-1 receptors binding properties, the atypical antipsychotic brexpiprazole shares many properties with aripiprazole. Brexpiprazole is currently being tested for its efficacy and safety in the treatment of agitation in patients with Alzheimer's disease (Porsteinsson and Antonsdottir, 2017).

Sleep–Wake Issues

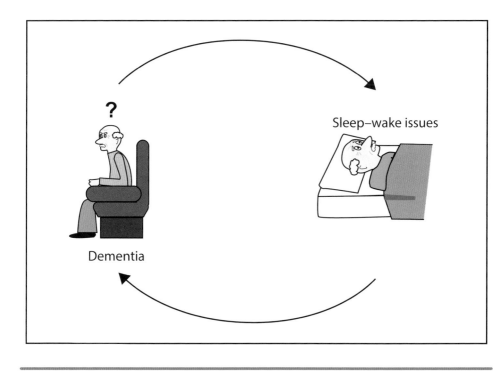

FIGURE 5.35. Insomnia is not an unavoidable consequence of getting older but is often seen in patients with dementia. Insomnia disrupts the critical balance of circadian rhythms and may also increase the risk for falls in elderly patients. Before initiating any pharmacological agent for sleep, it is important that attempts be made to rule out poor sleep hygiene, pain, urinary incontinence, or other conditions that may be contributing to sleep–wake issues. There are several pharmacological options for the treatment of insomnia; however, non-pharmacological options, including morning bright light therapy and cognitive behavioral therapy for insomnia, may be effective and should likely be tried first-line. Interestingly, not only are sleep–wake issues common in patients with dementia, circadian rhythm disruption may be a risk factor for dementia and appropriate treatment may lower dementia risk or improve cognitive performance in patients who have dementia (Schroek et al, 2016; Lanctot et al, 2017; Spira and Gottesman, 2017; McCleery et al, 2016).

Neurobiology of Sleep–Wake

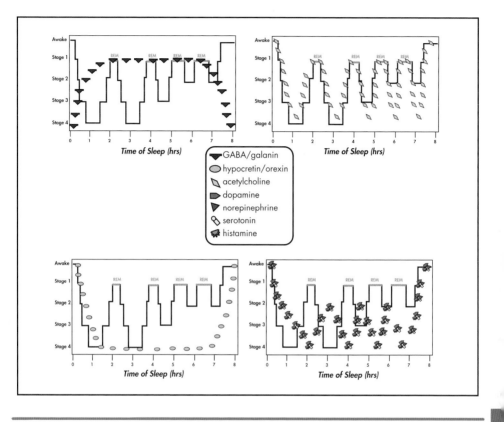

FIGURE 5.36. Neurotransmitters fluctuate on both a circadian (24-hour) basis as well as throughout the sleep cycle. GABA and galanin levels steadily increase during the first couple of hours of sleep, plateau, and then steadily decline before one wakes. Unlike GABA/galanin levels, hypocretin/orexin levels steadily decrease during the first couple of hours of sleep, plateau, and then steadily increase before one wakes. Acetylcholine levels fluctuate throughout the sleep cycle, reaching their lowest levels during stage 4 sleep and peaking during REM sleep. Dopamine, norepinephrine, serotonin, and histamine levels demonstrate a different trend. They peak during stage 2 sleep and are at their lowest during REM sleep. Treatments aimed at correcting sleep–wake issues seek to normalize deviations from these normal neurotransmitter fluctuations (Stahl and Morrissette, 2016).

Sleep–Wake Phase Advance

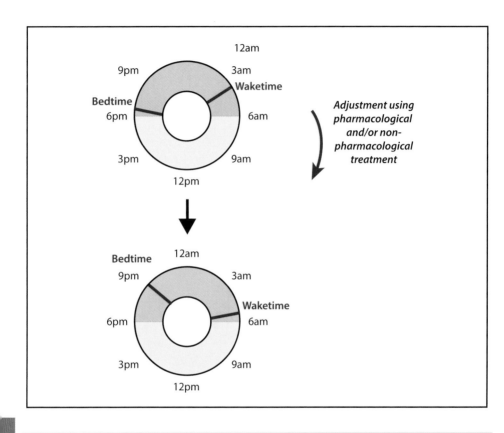

FIGURE 5.37. Many elderly patients with dementia have an advanced sleep–wake phase disorder (ASPD) in which they go to bed earlier and awaken earlier than desired, often by 4–6 hours outside of the typical sleep–wake cycle. There are several pharmacological and non-pharmacological strategies that may be effective for synchronizing the internal clock with external environmental and social cues. Adjusting this circadian clock may improve both insomnia and excessive daytime sleepiness. Treatments for ASPD include bright light therapy, chronobiotics (including melatonin, ramelteon, or tasimelteon), the stimulants armodafinil and modafinil (which hypothetically inhibit GABA and increase levels of dopamine, norepinephrine, histamine, and hypocretin/orexin), and structured sleep–wake schedules (Stahl and Morrissette, 2016).

Sundowning

Potential Causes
Degeneration of SCN
Decreased melatonin production
Impaired cholinergic input to SCN
HPA-axis dysregulation
Physiological/medical factors (hunger, body temperature, pain, etc.)
Environmental factors (end-of-day caregiver fatigue, noise, etc.)
Potential Treatments
Bright light therapy
Melatonin
Cholinesterase inhibitors
Minimize noise/stimulation
Avoid afternoon napping
Music therapy
Aromatherapy

FIGURE 5.38. Sundown syndrome, or sundowning, refers to the emergence or worsening of behavioral symptoms during the late afternoon/early evening when the sun goes down. As many as 66% of patients with dementia exhibit sundowning, with worsening of agitation, aggression, wandering, screaming, hallucinations, and confusion occurring around sunset and increasing the risk of institutionalization. There are several hypothesized neurobiological bases for sundowning but relatively limited treatment options. Although antipsychotics, benzodiazepines, and hypnotic agents are commonly prescribed for behavioral disturbances, these agents may actually worsen sundown syndrome (Canevelli et al, 2016).

HPA: hypothalamic–pituitary–adrenal; SCN: suprachiasmatic nucleus

Benzodiazepines

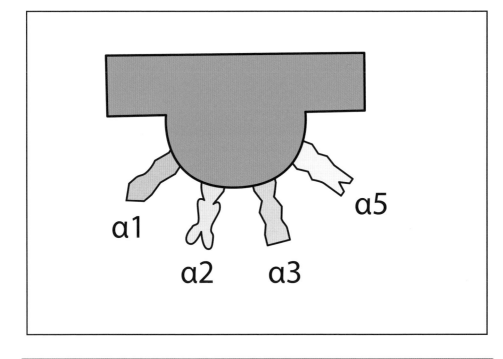

FIGURE 5.39. The benzodiazepine hypnotics all bind to α1, α2, α3, and α5 subunits of the GABA-A receptor. However, α subunit expression differs throughout the brain, and it is the selectivity for various α subunits that lends individual benzodiazepines their assorted effects outside of sedation (e.g., anxiolytic, anti-pain). All benzodiazepines carry a high risk of tolerance and withdrawal effects and are therefore not recommended for the long-term treatment of insomnia or agitation. Benzodiazepines are particularly not recommended in elderly patients with dementia as they may greatly increase the risk of falls, fractures, and death as well as worsening cognitive impairment (Stahl, 2013; Macfarlane and O'Connor, 2016; Preuss et al, 2016; Schroek et al, 2016; Torrisi et al, 2017; Gravielle, 2015).

Nonbenzodiazepine Hypnotics

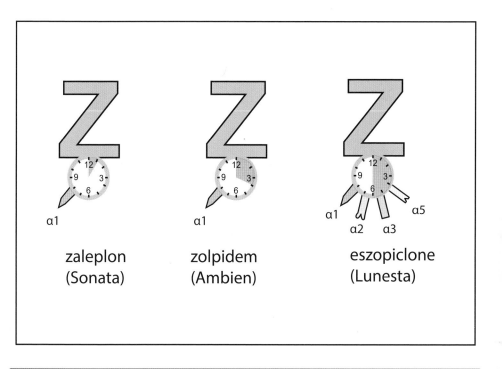

FIGURE 5.40. Unlike the benzodiazepine hypnotics, the non-benzodiazepine hypnotics (also known as "Z-drugs"), including zaleplon and zolpidem, bind selectively to 1 or 2 α subunits of the GABA-A receptor. The selectivity of non-benzodiazepines is hypothesized to underlie the non-sedative properties of individual agents. For example, binding to α2 and α3 subunits may impart anxiolytic, antidepressant, and anti-pain effects. Another Z-drug, eszopiclone, does not bind selectively; however, the binding of eszopiclone is different from that of benzodiazepine hypnotics. Therefore, Z-drugs are believed to carry less risk of tolerance than benzodiazepine hypnotics; in fact, eszopiclone is the only hypnotic agent approved for use over 35 days (Stahl, 2013).

Melatonin and Melatonin Agonists

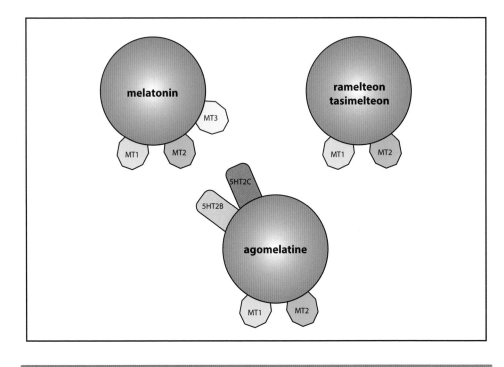

FIGURE 5.41. Endogenous melatonin is secreted by the pineal gland and mainly acts in the suprachiasmatic nucleus to regulate circadian rhythms. There are three types of receptors for melatonin: melatonin 1 and 2 (MT1 and MT2), which are both involved in sleep and circadian rhythms, and melatonin 3 (MT3), which is not thought to be involved in sleep physiology. When given at the appropriate time, melatonin (or a melatonin agonist such as ramelteon, tasimelteon, or agomelatine) may help promote sleep by resetting the sleep–wake cycle. Melatonin itself, available over the counter, acts at MT1 and MT2 receptors as well as at the melatonin 3 (MT3) site. Both ramelteon and tasimelteon are MT1 and MT2 receptor agonists and seem to improve sleep onset, though not necessarily sleep maintenance. Agomelatine is not only an MT1 and MT2 receptor agonist but also a 5HT2C and 5HT2B receptor antagonist; it is available as an antidepressant in Europe. Ramelteon is FDA-approved for the treatment of insomnia, and tasimelteon is FDA-approved for the treatment of Non-24-Hour Sleep–Wake disorder (Stahl, 2013; Bonacci et al, 2015; Shroek et al, 2016).

Hypocretin/Orexin

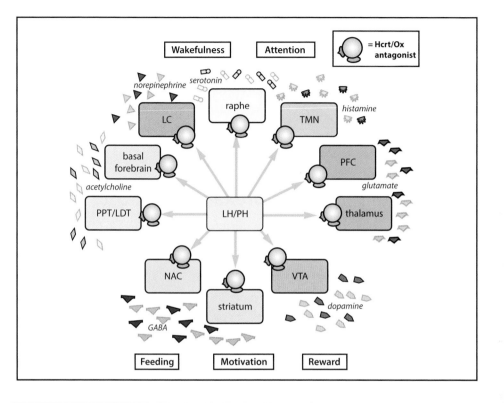

FIGURE 5.42. Hypocretin/orexins (Hcrt/Ox) have excitatory actions on various brain areas, stimulating the release of an assortment of neurotransmitters involved in wakefulness and arousal as well as feeding, motivation, and reward behaviors. The blockade of hypocretin/orexin receptors via Hcrt/Ox antagonists may therefore not only be useful for the treatment of insomnia (by reducing wakefulness) but may also have therapeutic value for the treatment of disorders of addiction, compulsivity, and overeating/obesity (Scammel and Winrow, 2011).

LC: locus coeruleus; NAC: nucleus accumbens; PFC: prefrontal cortex; PPT/LDT: pedunculopontine and laterodorsal tegmental nuclei; TMN: tuberomammillary nucleus; VTA: ventral tegmental area

Hypocretin/Orexin Antagonists

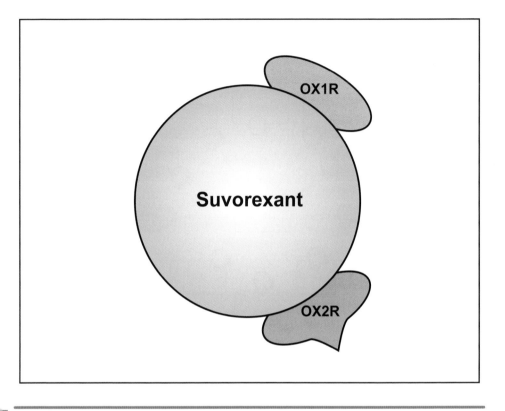

FIGURE 5.43. Given that hypocretin/orexin antagonists promote sleep without acting directly on GABA receptors, it is hypothesized that hypocretin/orexin antagonists will have fewer side effects than many earlier-generation hypnotics. The hypocretin/orexin antagonist, suvorexant, is approved for the treatment of insomnia and appears to promote sleep without causing rebound insomnia or risk of dependence (Shroek et al, 2016; Scammell and Winrow, 2011).

Modafinil/Armodafinil

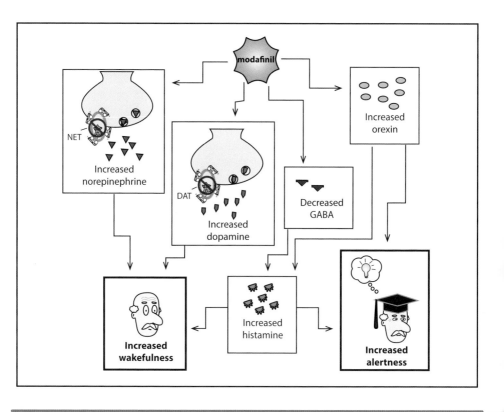

FIGURE 5.44. Modafinil and its R-enantiomer, armodafinil, increase both norepinephrine (NE) and dopamine (DA), possibly via their blockade of both the NE and DA reuptake transporters (NET and DAT, respectively). The actions of NE at alpha-adrenergic receptors and DA at dopamine D2 receptors are thought to contribute to the wake-promoting properties of modafinil. Orexin is a key component of the arousal system; thus, the hypothesized action of modafinil on the orexinergic system may help increase alertness. Additionally, modafinil may indirectly increase histamine, either by reducing GABAergic inhibition of histaminergic neurons or via actions at orexinergic neurons. The increase in histamine may contribute to both the wake-promoting effects of modafinil as well as the potential of modafinil to increase alertness (Stahl and Morrissette, 2016).

REM Sleep Behavior Disorder Treatment

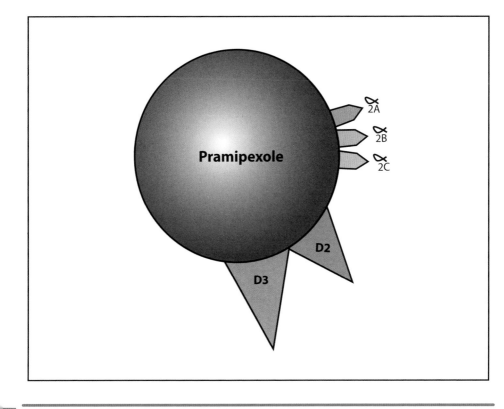

FIGURE 5.45. REM sleep behavior disorder (RSBD), which causes patients to "act out" their dreams, often occurs in the context of alpha-synucleinopathy dementias. In fact, 60% of patients presenting with RSBD are actually presenting with an early manifestation of dementia with Lewy bodies. The benzodiazepine, clonazepam, is often used to treat RSBD; however, given the risks associated with benzodiazepine use in patients with dementia, the dopamine D2/D3 receptor agonist pramipexole, which may also be efficacious, may be preferred in this patient population (Shroek et al, 2016; Torrisi et al, 2016).

Benefit vs. Harm of Psychotropic Treatment in Elderly Patients with Dementia

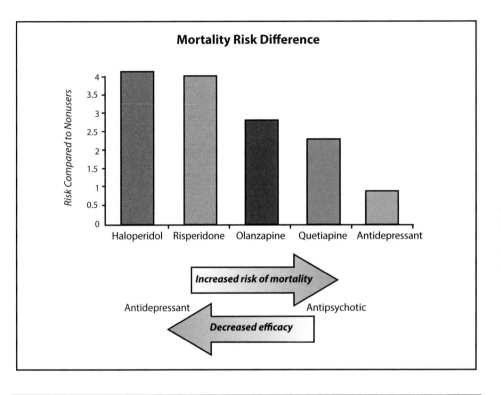

FIGURE 5.46. Although the treatment of secondary behavioral issues, including depression, psychosis, and agitation/aggression, is often deemed necessary for patients with dementia in order to delay institutionalization and improve quality of life for both patients and their caregivers, there is a fine balance between what will be safest vs. what will be effective. The antipsychotics (especially conventional, first-generation antipsychotics such as haloperidol) convey the greatest risk of mortality but may be the most effective agents for troublesome neuropsychiatric symptoms. Antidepressants have a more limited efficacy but are in many cases associated with less risk of mortality. Despite their lack of robust efficacy in this patient population, various psychotropics are still used quite often; alternative, non-pharmacological measures should always be first line in the treatment of neuropsychiatric symptoms in patients with dementia, and caution is warranted if the decision to initiate treatment with any psychotropic agent is made (Maust et al, 2015; van der Spek et al, 2016).

Treatment Considerations in Elderly Patients With Dementia

Contraindicated STOPP/START Criteria Applying to Psychotropic Medications
Phenothiazines should not be used
Anticholinergic or antimuscarinic agents should not be used in patients with dementia or delirium
Antipsychotics (except clozapine and quetiapine) should not be used in patients with Lewy body dementias
Benzodiazepines should not be used for more than 4 weeks
Use of two or more drugs with anticholinergic or antimuscarinic properties should be avoided
Tricyclic antidepressants should not be used
First-generation, conventional drugs should not be used
More than one medication from the hypnotic, sedative, antidepressant, anxiolytic, and antipsychotic class of medication should not be used

FIGURE 5.47. It has been estimated that approximately 60% of nursing home residents (undoubtedly many of whom have dementia) are prescribed unnecessary medications whereas 42% may not be getting potentially beneficial medications. This failure to properly utilize medications in the elderly population contributes to morbidity, mortality, and poor quality of life. Additionally, many geriatric patients, including those with dementia, are on numerous medications for a variety of physical, neurological, and psychological disorders. It is critical that potential drug interactions are considered before placing an elderly patient with dementia on a new medication, as the consequences of certain drug interactions can be fatal. A panel of experts has recently set forth the Screening Tool of Older Person's Prescriptions/Screening Tools to Alert Doctors to Right Treatment Medication Criteria (STOPP/START) guidelines to aid clinicians in the appropriate treatment of elderly patients, including those with dementia (Khodyakov et al, 2017; Levy and Collins, 2007; Norgaard et al, 2017).

Caregiver Care

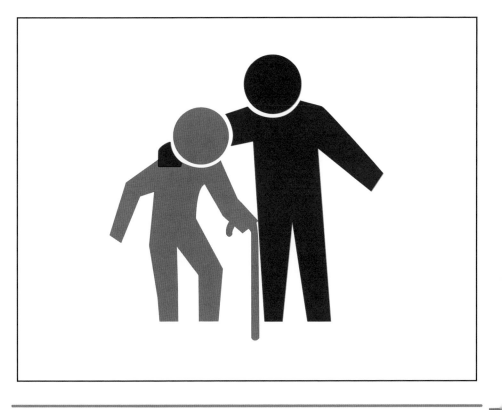

FIGURE 5.48. Providing round-the-clock care for a loved one with dementia can exact tremendous financial, emotional, mental, and physical consequences. Caring for an individual with dementia increases one's risk for numerous physical and psychological illnesses including depression, hypertension, and coronary heart disease. In the United States, the tasks required of a family caregiver, from bathing, toileting, dressing, and feeding the patient, are estimated to be valued at a contribution to the nation of approximately $221 billion. While the role of the clinician is typically focused on the patient with dementia, recommendations are now stressing the importance of also assessing caregiver well-being (using instruments such as the Zariit Burden Interview and the Caregiver Strain Index) and steering caregivers toward valuable support resources such as the Alzheimer's Association and the National Family Caregiver Support Program (Gitlin and Hodgson, 2016; Jennings et al, 2017; Alzheimer's Association, 2017).

The genetics, neuropathology, and clinical presentation is complex, diverse, and often overlapping among the various types of dementias. However, differential diagnosis is critical. Although disease-modifying treatments for virtually all forms of non-reversible dementias have yet to be discovered, an accurate differential diagnosis is key in order to design clinical trials aimed at discovering novel treatments for different causes of dementia. Additionally, the use of certain neuroleptics may have some benefit (albeit limited) in select dementias (e.g., cholinesterase inhibitors for Alzheimer's disease) but may be ineffective and possibly contraindicated in other dementias (e.g., cholinesterase inhibitors in frontotemporal lobar degeneration disorders). The understanding of the complex diagnosis and neurobiological substrates underlying each form of dementia is critical to the effective management of patients as well as the development of potential disease-modifying treatments and lifestyle strategies aimed at reducing one's risk of developing dementia.

Alafuzoff I, Hartikainen P. Alpha-synucleinopathies. Handbook of Clinical Neurology 2017; 145:339–353.

Albert MS, Dekosky ST, Dickson D et al. The diagnosis of mild cognitive impairments due to Alzheimer's disease: recommendations from the National Institute on Aging–Alzheimer's Association workgroups on diagnostic guidelines for Alzheimer's disease. Alzheimer's Dement 2011;7(3):270–9.

Alexopoulos GS, Abrams RC, Young RC et al. Cornell Scale for Depression in Dementia. Biol Psychiatry 1988;23:271–84.

Alexopoulos P, Werle L, Roesler J et al. Conflicting cerebrospinal fluid biomarkers and progression to dementia due to Alzheimers disease. Alz Res Ther 2016;8:51.

Allan CL, Behrman S, Ebmeier KP et al. Diagnosing early cognitive decline — when, how, and for whom? Maturitas 2017;96:103–8.

Alzheimer's Association. Alzheimer's disease facts and figures. Alzheimers Dement 2017;13:325–73.

Amar BR, Yadav R, Janardhan Reddy YC et al. A clinical profile of patients with Parkinson's disease and psychosis. Ann Indian Acad Neurol 2014;17(20):187–92.

Anand K, Sabbagh M. Amyloid imaging: poised for integration into medical practice. Neurotherapeutics 2017;14(1):54–61.

Anand R, Kaushal A, Wani WY et al. Road to Alzheimer's disease: the pathomechanism underlying. Pathobiology 2012;72(2):55–71.

Anang JB, Gagnon JF, Bertrand JA et al. Predictors of dementia in Parkinson's disease: a prospective cohort study. Neurology 2014;83(14):1253.

Anastasiou CA, Yannakoulia M, Kosmidis MH et al. Mediterranean diet and cognitive health: initial results from the Hellenic Longitudinal Investigation of ageing and diet. PLOS ONE 2017;12(8):e0182048.

Annus A, Csati A, Vecsei L. Prion diseases: new considerations. Clin Neurology Neurosurg 2016;150:125–32.

Arai T. Significance and limitation of the pathological classification of TDP-43 proteinopathy. Neuropathology 2014;34(6):578–88.

Arbor SC, LaFontaine M, Cumbay M. Amyloid-beta Alzheimer targets— protein processing, lipid rafts, and amyloid-beta pores. Yale J Biol Med 2016;89:5–21.

Arendt T, Steiler JT, Holzer M. Tau and tauopathies. Brain Res Bull 2016;126:238–92.

Aridi YS, Walker JL, Wright ORL. The association between the Mediterranean dietary pattern and cognitive health: a systematic review. Nutrients 2017;9(7):E674.

Asken BM, Sullan MJ, Snyder AR et al. Factors influencing clinical correlates of chronic traumatic encephalopathy (CTE): a review. Neuropsychol Rev 2016;26:340–63.

Atri A. Imaging of neurodegenerative cognitive and behavioral disorders: practical considerations for dementia clinical practice. Handb Clin Neurol 2016;136:971–84.

Atri A, Frolich L, Ballard C et al. Effect of idalopirdine as adjunct to cholinesterase inhibitors on change in cognition in patients with Alzheimer disease: three randomized clinical trials. JAMA 2018;319(2):130–42.

Atwood CS, Bishop GM, Perry G et al. Amyloid-beta: a vascular sealant that protects against hemorrhage? J Neurosci Rev 2002;4(3):203–14.

Atwood CS, Robinson SR, Smith MA. Amyloid-beta: redox-metal chelator and antioxidant. J Alzheimers Dis 2002b;4(3):203–14.

Azizi SA, Azizi SA. Synucleinopathies in neurodegenerative diseases: accomplices, an inside job and selective vulnerability. Neurosci Letters 2018;672:150–2.

Ballard C et al. Dementia in Down's syndrome. Lancet Neurol 2016;15:622–36.

Ballard C, Khan Z, Clack H et al. Nonpharmacological treatment of Alzheimer disease. Can J Psychiatry 2011;56(10):589–95.

Ballard C, Neill D, O'Brien J, et al. Anxiety, depression and psychosis in vascular dementia: prevalence and associations. J Affect Disord 2000;59(2):97–106.

Ballard C, Oyebode F. Psychotic symptoms in patients with dementia. Int J Geriatr Psychiatry 1995;10(9):743–52.

Bao AM, Meynen G, Swaab DF. The stress system in depression and neurodegeneration: focus on the human hypothalamus. Brain Res Rev 2008;57(2):531–53.

Bassetti CL, Bargiotas P. REM sleep behavior disorder. Front Neurol Neurosci 2018;41:104–16.

Bennett S, Thomas AJ. Depression and dementia: cause, consequence or coincidence? Maturita 2014;79:184–90.

Benskey MJ, Perez RG, Manfredsson FP. The contribution of alpha synuclein to neuronal survival and function—implications for Parkinson's disease. J Neurochemistry 2016;137:331–59.

Bluml V, Regier MD, Hlavin G et al. Lithium in the public water supply and suicide mortality in Texas. J Psychiatr Res 2013;47(3):407–11.

Bonacci JM, Venci JV, Ghandi MA. Tasimelteon (Hetlioz®): a new melatonin receptor agonist for the treatment of non-24 sleep-wake disorder. J Pharm Pract 2015;28(5):473–8.

Bonifacio G, Zamboni G. Brain imaging in dementia. Postgrad Med J 2016;92:333–40.

Boxer AL, Yu JT, Golbe LI et al. Advances in progressive supranuclear palsy: new diagnostic criteria, biomarkers, and therapeutic approaches. Lancet Neurol 2017;166:552–63.

Braak H, Del Tredici K, Rub U et al. Staging of brain pathology related to sporadic Parkinson's disease. Neurobiol Aging 2003;24(2):197–211.

Bronzuoli MR, Iacomino A, Steardo L et al. Targeting neuroinflammation in Alzheimer's disease. J Inflamm Res 2016;9:199–208.

Buoli M, Serati M, Caldiroli A et al. Pharmacological management of psychiatric symptoms in frontotemporal dementia: a systematic review. J Geriatr Psychiatry 2017;30(3):162–9.

Burchell JT, Panegyres PK. Prion diseases: immunotargets and therapy. ImmunoTargets Ther 2016;5:57–68.

Burmester B, Leathem J, Merrick P. Subjective cognitive complaints and objective cognitive function in aging: a systematic review and meta-analysis of recent cross-sectional findings. Neuropsychol Rev 2016;26:376–93.

Burns A, Jacoby R, Levy R. Psychiatric phenomena in Alzheimer's disease. II: Disorders of perception. Br J Psychiatry 1990;157:76–81, 92–4.

Canevelli M, Valleta M, Trebbastoni A et al. Sundowning in dementia: clinical relevance, pathophysiological determinants, and therapeutic approaches. Front Med (Lausanne) 2016;3:73.

Caraci F, Copani A, Nicoletti F et al. Depression and Alzheimer's disease: neurobiological links and common pharmacological targets. Eur J Pharmacol 2010;626(1):64–71.

Cardenas-Aguayo, M. del C. Physiological role of amyloid beta in neural cells: the cellular trophic activity. In Heinbockel T, ed. Neurochemistry. InTech Open Access Publisher, 2014; doi:10.5772/57398.

Cederholm T. Fish consumption and omega-3 fatty acid supplementation for prevention or treatment of cognitive decline, dementia or Alzheimer's disease in older adults—any news? Curr Opin Clin Nutr Metab Care 2017;20;104–9.

Cepoiu-Martin M, Tam-Tham H, Patten S et al. Predictors of long-term care placement in persons with dementia: a systematic review and meta-analysis. Int J Geriatr Psychiatry 2016;31:1151–71.

Chakraborty A, de Wit NM, van der Flier WM et al. The blood brain barrier in Alzheimer's disease. Vasc Pharmacol 2017;89:12–18.

Cheston R, Ivanecka A. Individual and group psychotherapy with people diagnosed with dementia: a systematic review of the literature. Geriatr Psychiatry 2017;32:3–31.

Cheung CY, Ikram MK, Chen C et al. Imaging retina to study dementia and stroke. Prog Brain Retinal Eye Res 2017;57:89–107.

Chutinet A, Rost NS. White matter disease as a biomarker for long-term cerebrovascular disease and dementia. Curr Treat Options Cardiovasc Med 2014;16(3):292.

Cohen-Mansfield J, Billig N. Agitated behaviors in the elderly. I. A conceptual review. J Am Geriatr Soc 1986;34(1):711–21.

Corcoran C, Wong ML, O'Keane V. Bupropion in the management of apathy. J Psychopharm 2004;18(1):133–5.

Cummings J. Alzheimer's disease: clinical trials and the amyloid hypothesis. Ann Acad Med Singapore 2011;40(7):304–6.

Cummings JL, Lyketsos CG, Peskind ER et al. Effect of dextromethorphan-quinidine on agitation in patients with Alzheimer's disease dementia: a randomized clinical trial. JAMA 2015;314(12):1242–54.

Delgado-Morales R, Esteller M. Opening up the DNA methylome of dementia. Mol Psychiatr 2017;22(4):485–496.

Dennis M, Shine L, John A et al. Risk of adverse outcomes for older people with dementia prescribed antipsychotic medication: a population based e-cohort study. Neurol Ther 2017;6:5777.

Depypere H, Vierin A, Weyers S et al. Alzheimer's disease, apolipoprotein E and hormone replacement therapy. Maturitas 2016;94:98–105.

DeSimone CV, Graff-Radford J, El-Harasis MA et al. Cerebral amyloid angiopathy: diagnosis, clinical implications, and management strategies in atrial fibrillation. J Am Coll Cardiol 2017;70:1173–82.

Deutschlander AB, Ross OA, Dickson DW et al. Atypical parkinsonism syndromes: a general neurologist's perspective. Eur J Neurol 2018;25(1):41–58.

Ducharme S, Price BH, Dickerson BC. Apathy: a neurocircuitry model based on frontotemporal dementia. J Neural Neurosurg Psychiatry 2018;89:389–96.

Dugger BN, Dickson DW. Pathology of neurodegenerative diseases. Cold Springs Harb Perspect Biol 2017;9(7):a028035.

Eddy CM, Parkinson EG, Rickards HE. Changes in mental state and behavior in Huntington's disease. Lancet Psychiatry 2016;3:1079–86.

Emre M. Treatment of dementia associated with Parkinson's disease. Parkinsonism Relat Disord 2007;13 (Suppl 3):S457–61.

Eusebio A, Koric L, Felician O et al. Progressive supranuclear palsy and corticobasal degeneration: diagnostic challenges and clinicopathological considerations. Rev Neurol (Paris) 2016;172(8–9):488–502.

Evan C, Weintraub D. Case for and against specificity of depression in Alzheimer's disease. Psychiatry Clin Neurosci 2010;64(4):358–66.

Fajardo VA, Fajardo VA, LeBlanc PJ et al. Examining the relationship between trace lithium in drinking water and the rising rates of age-adjusted Alzheimer's disease mortality in Texas. J Alzheimers Dis 2018;61(1):425–34.

Fan LY, Chiu MJ. Pharmacological treatment for Alzheimer's disease: current approaches and future strategies. Acta Neurol Taiwan 2010;19(4):228–45.

Farhadian S, Patel P, Spudich S. Neurological complications of HIC infection. Currr Infect Dis Rep 2017;19:50.

Farina N, Morrell L, Banerjee S. What is the therapeutic value of antidepressants in dementia? A narrative review. Geriatr Psychiatry 2017;32:32–49.

Fernandez-Matarrubia M, Matias-Guiu JA, Cabrera-Martin MN et al. Different apathy clinical profile and neural correlates in behavioral variant frontotemporal dementia and Alzheimer's disease. Int J Geriatr Psychiatry 2018;33:141–50.

Fernandez-Matarrubia M, Matias-Guiu JA, Moreno-Ramos Tet al. Validation of the Lille's Apathy Rating Scale in very mild to moderate dementia. Am J Geriatr Psychiatry 2016;24(7):517–27.

Ferrero H, Solas M, Francis PT et al. Serotonin 5-HT6 receptor antagonists in Alzheimer's disease: therapeutic rationale and current development status. CNS Drugs 2017;31:19–32.

Foo H, Mak E, Yong TT. Progression of subcortical atrophy in mild Parkinson's disease and its impact on cognition. Eur J Neurol 2017;24(2):341–8.

Ford AH. Preventing delirium in dementia: managing risk factors. Maturitas 2016;92:35–40.

Ford AH, Almeida OP. Management of depression in patients with dementia: is pharmacological treatment justified? Drugs Aging 2017;34:89–95.

Forman MS, Trojanowski JQ, Lee VM. TDP-43: a novel neurodegenerative proteinopathy. Curr Opin Neurobiol 2007;17(5):548–55.

Fraker J, Kales HC, Blazek M, The role of the occupational therapist in the management of neuropsychiatric symptoms of dementia in clinical settings. Occup Ther Health Care 2014;28(1):4–20.

Galvin JE. Improving the clinical detection of Lewy body dementia with the Lewy Body Composite Risk Score. Alzheimers Dement (Amst) 2015;1(3):316–24.

Garay RP, Grossberg GT. AVP-786 for the treatment of agitation in dementia of the Alzheimer's type. Exp Opin Invest Drugs 2017;26(1):121–32.

Gass J, Prudencio M, Stetler C et al. Progranulin: an emerging target for FTLD therapies. Brain Res 2012;1462:118–28.

Geerlings MI, den Hijer T, Koudstaal PJ et al. History of depression, depressive symptoms, and medial temporal lobe atrophy and the risk of Alzheimer's disease. Neurology 2008;70(15):1258–64.

Gehres SW, Rocha A, Leuzy A et al. Cognitive intervention as an early non-pharmacological strategy in Alzheimer's disease: a translational perspective. Front Aging Neurosci 2016;8(280):1–4.

Geldmacher DS, Provenano G, McRae T et al. Donepezil is associated with delayed nursing home placement in patients with Alzheimer's disease. J Am Geriatr Soc 2003;51(7):937–44.

Giri M, Zhang M, Lu Y. Genes associated with Alzheimer's disease: an overview and current status. Clin Interv Aging 2016;11:665–81.

Gitlin LN, Hodgson NA. Who should assess the needs of and care for a dementia patient's caregiver? AMA J Ethics 2016;18(12):1171–81.

Godyn J, Jonczyk J, Panek D et al. Therapeutic strategies for Alzheimer's disease in clinical trials. Pharmacol Rep 2016;68(1):127–38.

Goetz CG, Emre M, Dubois B. Parkinson's disease dementia: definitions, guidelines, and research perspectives in diagnosis. Ann Neurol 2008;64 (Suppl 2):S81–92.

Goldman JG, Holden S. Treatment of psychosis and dementia in Parkinson's disease. Curr Treat Options Neurol 2014;16(3):281.

Goodarzi Z, Mele B, Guo S et al. Guidelines for dementia or Parkinson's disease with depression or anxiety: a systematic review. BMC Neurology 2016;16(1):244.

Goodman RA, Lochner KA, Thambisetty M et al. Prevalence of dementia subtypes in United States Medicare fee-for-service beneficiaries, 2011-2013. Alzheimers Dement 2017;13:28–37.

Gordon E, Rohrer JD, Fox NC. Advances in neuroimaging in frontotemporal dementia. J Neurochem 2016;138(Suppl 1):193–210.

Grandy JK. Updated guidelines for the diagnosis of Alzheimer disease: a clinical review. JAAPA 2012;25(4):50–5.

Gravielle MC. Activation-induced regulation of GABAA receptors: is there a link with the molecular basis of benzodiazepine tolerance? Pharmacol Res 2016;109:92–100.

Gray SL, Hanlon JT. Anticholinergic medication use and dementia: latest evidence and clinical implications. Ther Adv Drug Saf 2016;7(5):217–24.

Greenberg SM, Charidimou A. Diagnosis of cerebral amyloid angiopathy: evolution of the Boston Criteria. Stroke 2018;49:491–7.

Gu Y, Brickman AM, Stern Y et al. Mediterranean diet and brain structure in a multiethnic elderly cohort. Neurology 2015;85(20):1744–51.

Gurnani AS, Gavett BE. The differential effects of Alzheimer's disease and Lewy body pathology on cognitive performance: a meta-analysis. Neuropsychol Rev 2017;27:1–17.

Hacksell U, Burstein ES, McFarland K et al. On the discovery and development of pimavanserin: a novel drug candidate for Parkinson's disease. Neurochem Res 2014;39(10):2008–17.

Hardman RJ, Kennedy G, Macpherson H et al. Adherence to a Mediterranean-style diet and effects on cognition in adults: a qualitative evaluation and systematic review of longitudinal and prospective trials. Front Nutr 2016;3(22):1–13.

Harper L, Barkhof F, Scheltens P et al. An algorithmic approach to structural imaging in dementia. J Neurol Neurosurg Psychiatry 2014;85(6):692–8.

Harrison JR, Owen MJ. Alzheimer's disease: the amyloid hypothesis on trial. Br J Psychiatry 2016;208(1):1–3.

Hasegawa M, Nonaka T, Masuda-Suzukake M. Prion-like mechanisms and potential therapeutic targets in neurodegenerative disorders. Pharmacol Ther 2017;172:22–33.

Herrmann N, Chau Sa, Kircanski I et al. Current and emerging treatment options for Alzheimer's disease: a systematic review. Drugs 2011;71(15):2031–65.

Herukka SK, Simonsen AH, Andreasen N et al. Recommendations for CSF AD biomarkers in the diagnostic evaluation of MCI. Alzeimers Dement 2017;13(3):285–95.

Hinz FI, Geschwind DH. Molecular genetics of neurodegenerative dementias. Cold Spring Harb Perspect Biol 2017;9:pii:a023705.

Hithersay R, Hamburg S, Knight B et al. Cognitive decline and dementia in Down syndrome. Curr Opin Psychiatry 2017;30(2):102–7.

Hongisto K, Hallikainen I, Seldander et al. Quality of Life in relation to neuropsychiatric symptoms in Alzheimer's disease: 5-year prospective ALSOVA cohort study. Int J Geriatr Psychiatry 2018;33(1):47–57.

Ince PG, Perry EK, Morris CM. Dementia with Lewy bodies: a distinct non-Alzheimer dementia syndrome? Brain Pathology 1998;8:299–324.

Jack Jr CR, Wiste HJ, Weigland SD et al. Defining imaging biomarker cut point for brain aging and Alzheimer's disease. Alzheimers Dement 2017;13(3):205–16.

Jellinger KA. Dementia with Lewy bodies and Parkinson's disease-dementia: current concepts and controversies. J Neural Transmission 2018;125(4):615–50.

Jena A, Renjen PN, Taneja S et al. Integrated (18)F-fluorodeoxyglucose positron emission tomography magnetic resonance imaging (^{18}F-FDG PET/MRI), a multimodality approach for comprehensive evaluation of dementia patients: a pictorial essay. Indian J Radiol Imaging 2015;25(4):342–52.

Jennings LA, Palimaru A, Corona MG et al. Patient and caregiver goals for dementia care. Qual Life Res 2017;26(3):685–93.

Johnson BP, Westlake KP. Link between Parkinson disease and rapid eye movement sleep behavior disorder with dream enactment: possible implications for early rehabilitation. Arch Phys Med Rehab 2018; 99:410–15.

Johnson DK, Watts AS, Chapin BA et al. Neuropsychiatric profiles in dementia. Alzheimer Dis Assoc Disord 2011;25(4):326–32.

Jonsson T, Atwal JK, Steinberg S et al. A mutation in APP protects against Alzheimer's disease and age-related cognitive decline. Nature 2012;488(7409):96–9.

Kapasi A, DeCarli C, Schneider JA. Impact of multiple pathologies on the threshold for clinically overt dementia. Acta Neuropathol 2017;134:171–86.

Karantzoulis S, Galvin JE. Distinguishing Alzheimer's disease from other major forms of dementia. Expert Rev Neurother 2011;11(11):1579–91.

Kertesz A, Munoz DG. Frontotemporal dementia. Med Clin North Am 2002;86(3):501–18.

Kessing LV, Sondergard L, Forman JL et al. Antidepressants and dementia. J Affect Disord 2009;117(1–2):24–9.

Khodyakov D, Ochoa A, Olivieri-Mui BL et al. Screening tool of older person's prescriptions/screening tools to alert doctors to right treatment medication criteria modified for U.S. nursing home setting. JAGS 2017;65:586–91.

Knight A, Bryan J, Murphy K. Is the Mediterranean diet a feasible approach to preserving cognitive function and reducing risk of dementia for older adults in Western countries? New insights and future directions. Ageing Res Rev 2016;25:85–101.

Knopman DS, Kramer JH, Boeve BF et al. Development of methodology for conducting clinical trials in frontotemporal lobar degeneration. Brain 2008;131(Pt 11):2957–68.

Kobylecki C, Jones M, Thompson JC et al. Cognitive-behavioural features of progressive supranuclear palsy syndrome overlap with frontotemporal dementia. J Neurol 2015;262:916–22.

Kok RM, Reynolds CF. Management of depression in older adults: a review. JAMA 2017;317(2):2114–22.

Kokjohn TA, Maarouf CL, Roher AE. Is Alzheimer's disease amyloidosis a result of a repair mechanism gone astray? Alzheimers Dement 2012;8(6):574–83.

Kolb HC, Andres JI. Tau positron emission tomography imaging. Cold Spring Harb Perspect Biol 2017;9(5):a023721.

Kong EH. Agitation in dementia: concept clarification. J Adv Nurs 2005;52(5):526–36.

Koronyo Y, Biggs D, Barron E et al. Retinal amyloid pathology and proof-of-concept imaging trial in Alzheimer's disease. JCI Insight 2017;2(16):93621.

Kovari E, Herrmann FR, Hof PR et al. The relationship between cerebral amyloid angiopathy and cortical microinfarcts in brain ageing and Alzheimer's disease. Neuropathol Appl Neurobiol 2013;39(5):498–509.

Kullmann S, Heni M, Hallschmid M et al. Brain insulin resistance at the crossroads of metabolic and cognitive disorders in humans. Physiol Rev 2016;96:1169–1209.

Kumar DK, Eimer WA, Tanzi RE et al. Alzheimer's disease: the potential therapeutic role of the natural antibiotic amyloid-B peptide. Neurodegener Dis Manag 2016;6(5):345–8.

Kumfor F, Zhen A, Hodges JR et al. Apathy in Alzheimer's disease and frontotemporal dementia: distinct clinical profiles and neural correlates. Cortex 2018;103:350–9.

Lanctot KL, Amatniek J, Ancoli-Isreal et al. Neuropsychiatric signs and symptoms of Alzheimer's disease: new treatment paradigms. Alz Dem Transl Res Clin Interv 2017;3:440–9.

Landin-Romero R, Tan R, Hodges HR et al. An update on semantic dementia: genetics, imaging, and pathology. Alz Res Ther 2016;8(1):52.

Larson EB, Wang L, Bowen JD et al. Exercise is associated with reduced risk for incident dementia among persons 65 years of age and older. Ann Intern Med 2006;144(2):73–81.

Lee HS, Park SW, Park YJ. Effects of physical activity programs on the improvement of dementia symptom: a meta-analysis. Biomed Res Int 2016;2016:2920146.

Lee SH, Zabolotny JM, Huang H et al. Insulin in the nervous system and the mind: functions in metabolism, memory, and mood. Mol Metab 2016;5:589–601.

Leroi I, Voulgari A, Breitner JC et al. The epidemiology of psychosis in dementia. Am J Geriatr Psychiatry 2003;11(1):83–91.

Levy RH, Collins C. Risk and predictability of drug interactions in the elderly. Int Rev Neurobio 2007;81:235–51.

Li Y, Li Y, Li X et al. Head injury as a risk factor for dementia and Alzheimer's disease: a systematic review and meta-analysis of 32 observational studies. PLOS ONE 2017;12(1):e0169650.

Li Y, Sekine T, Funayama M et al. Clinicogenetic study of GBA mutations in patients with familial Parkinson's disease. Neurobiol Aging 2014;35(4):935.e3-8.

Lieberman A, Deep A, Shi J et al. Downward finger displacement distinguishes Parkinson disease dementia from Alzheimer disease. Int J Neurosci 2018;128(2):151–4.

Lim JK, Li QX, He Z et al. The eye as a biomarker for Alzheimer's disease. Front Neurosci 2016;10(536):1–14.

Lim SY, Kim EJ, Kim A et al. Nutritional factors affecting mental health. Clin Nutr Res 2016;5(3):143–52.

Ling H. Clinical approach to progressive supranuclear palsy. J Mov Disord 2016;9(1):3–13.

Lippmann S, Perugula ML. Delirium or dementia? Innov Clin Neurosci 2016;13(9–10):56–7.

Liscic RM, Srulijes K, Groger A et al. Differentiation of progressive supranuclear palsy: clinical, imaging and laboratory tools. Acta Neurol Scand 2013;127:361–70.

Llorens F, Karch A, Golanska E et al. Cerebrospinal fluid biomarker-based diagnosis of sporadic Creutzfeldt-Jakob Disease: a validation study for previously established cutoffs. Dement Geriatr Cogn Disord 2017;43:71–80.

Lochhead JD, Nelson MA, Maguire GA. The treatment of behavioral disturbances and psychosis associated with dementia. Psychiatr Pol 2016;50(2):311–22.

Lopez OL, Becker JT, Sweet RA et al. Psychiatric symptoms vary with the severity of dementia in probable Alzheimer's disease. J Neuropsychiatry Clin Neurosci 2003;15(3):346–53.

Lyketsos CG, Carillo MC, Ryan JM et al. Neuropsychiatric symptoms in Alzheimer's disease. Alzheimers Dement 2011;7(5):532–9.

Lyketsos CG, Lopez O, Jones B et al. Prevalence of neuropsychiatric symptoms in dementia and mild cognitive impairment: results from the cardiovascular health study. JAMA 2002;288(12):1475–83.

Lyketsos CG, Steinberg M, Tschanz JT et al. Mental and behavioral disturbances in dementia: findings from the Cache County Study on Memory in Aging. Am J Psychiatry 2000;157(5):704–7.

Macfarlane S, O'Connor D. Managing behavioural and psychological symptoms in dementia. Aust Prescr 2016;39:123–5.

Mackenzie IR, Neumann M. Molecular neuropathology of frontotemporal dementia: insights into disease mechanisms from postmortem studies. J Neurochem 2016;138(Suppl 1):54–70.

Mackenzie IR, Munoz DG, Kusaka H et al. Distinct subtypes of FTLD-FUS. Acta Neuropathol 2011;121(2):207–18.

MacLeod R, Hillert EK, Cameron RT et al. The role and therapeutic targeting of α-, β-, and g-secretase in Alzheimer's disease. Future Sci OA 2015;1(3):FSO11.

Mallik A, Drzezga, Minoshima S. Clinical amyloid imaging. Semin Nucl Med 2017;47:31–43.

Maloney B, Lahiri DK. Epigenetics of dementia: understanding the disease as a transformation rather than a state. Lancet Neurol 2016;15:760–74.

Marcason W. What are the components of the MIND diet? J Acad Nutr Diet 2015;115(10):1744.

Marciani DJ. Alzheimer's disease vaccine development: a new strategy focusing on immune modulation. J Neuroimmunol 2015;287:54–63.

Marin RS, Fogel BS, Hawkins J et al. Apathy: a treatable symptom. J Neuropsychiatry 1995;7:23–30.

Maust DT, Kim HM, Seyfried LS et al. Antipsychotics, other psychotropics, and the risk of death in patients with dementia: number needed to harm. JAMA Psychiatry 2015;72(5):438–45.

McCarter S, St Louis EK, Boeve BF. Sleep disturbances in frontotemporal dementia. Curr Neurol Neurosci Rep 2016;16:85.

McCleery J, Cohen DA, Sharpley AL. Pharmacotherapies for sleep disturbances in dementia (review). Cochrane Database System Rev 2016;11:CD009178.

McGirt MJ, Woodworth G, Coon AL et al. Diagnosis, treatment, and analysis of long-term outcomes in idiopathic normal-pressure hydrocephalus. Neurosurgery 2005;57(4):699–705.

McKeith IG, Dickson DW, Lowe J et al. Diagnosis and management of dementia with Lewy bodies: third report of the DLB consortium. Neurology 2005;65(12):1863–72.

Mendiola-Precoma J, Berumen LC, Padilla K et al. Therapies for prevention and treatment of Alzheimer's disease. BioMed Res Int 2016; 2016:2589276.

Meyer PT, Frings L, Rucker G et al. 18F-FDG PET in Parkinsonism: differential diagnosis and evaluation of cognitive impairment. J Nucl Med 2017;58(12):1888–98.

Michel J-P. Is it possible to delay or prevent age-related cognitive decline? Korean J Fam Med 2016;37:263–6.

Mioshi E, Flanagan E, Knopman D. Detecting change with the CDR-FTLD: differences between FTLD and AD dementia. Int J Geriatr Psychiatry 2017;32(9):977–82.

Mioshi E, Hsieh S, Savage S et al. Clinical staging and disease progression in frontotemporal dementia. Neurology 2010;74(20):1591–7.

Montenigro PH, Baugh CM, Daneshvar DH et al. Clinical subtypes of chronic traumatic encephalopathy: literature review and proposed research diagnostic criteria for traumatic encephalopathy syndrome. Alz Res Ther 2014;6:68.

Moraros J, Nwankwo C, Patten SB et al. The association of antidepressant drug usage with cognitive impairment or dementia, including Alzheimer disease: a systematic review and meta-analysis. Depress Anxiety 2017;34(3):217–26.

Mossello E, Boncinelli M, Caleri V et al. Is antidepressant treatment associated with reduced cognitive decline in Alzheimer's disease? Dement Geriatr Cogn Disord 2008;25(4):372–9.

Nalbandian A, Donkervoort S, Dec E et al. The multiple faces of valosin-containing protein-associated diseases: inclusion body myopathy with Paget's disease of bone, frontotemporal dementia, and amyotrophic lateral sclerosis. J Mol Neurosci 2011;45(3):522–31.

Ngandu T, Lehtisalo J, Solomon A et al. A 2 year multidomain intervention of diet, exercise, cognitive training, and vascular risk monitoring versus control to prevent cognitive decline in at-risk elderly people (FINGER): a randomized controlled trial. Lancet 2015;385:2255–63.

Noe E, Marder K, Bell KL et al. Comparison of dementia with Lewy bodies to Alzheimer's disease and Parkinson's disease with dementia. Movement Disorders 2004;19(1):60–7.

Norgaard A, Jensen-Dahm C, Gasse C et al. Psychotropic polypharmacy in patients with dementia: prevalence and predictors. J Alz Dis 2017;56(2):707–16.

O'Donnell CA, Browne S, Pierce M et al. Reducing dementia risk by targeting modifiable risk factors in mid-life: study protocol for the Innovative Midlife Intervention for Dementia Deterrence (In-MINDD) randomized controlled feasibility trial. Pilot Feasibility Studies 2015;1:40.

Ohta Y, Darwish M, Hishikawa N et al. Therapeutic effects of drug switching between acetylcholinesterase inhibitors in patients with Alzheimer's disease. Geriatr Gerontol Int 2017;17(11):1843–8.

Olszewska DA, Lonergan R, Fallon EM et al. Genetics of frontotemporal dementia. Curr Neurol Neurosci Rep 2016;16:107.

Pandya SY, Clem MA, Silva LM et al. Does mild cognitive impairment always lead to dementia? A review. J Neurol Sci 2016;369:58–62.

Panza F, Solfrizzi V, Seripa D et al. Tau-centric targets and drugs in clinical development for the treatment of Alzheimer's disease. BioMed Res Int 2016;2016:3245935.

Paoli RA, Botturi A, Ciammola A et al. Neuropsychiatric burden in Huntington's disease. Brain Sci 2017;7:67.

Park HK, Park KH, Yoon B et al. Clinical characteristics of parkinsonism in frontotemporal dementia according to subtypes. J Neurol Sci 2017;372:51–6.

Pascoal TA, Mathotaarachchi S, Shin M et al. Synergistic interaction between amyloid and tau predicts the progression to dementia. Alzheimers Dement 2017;13(6):644–53.

Pepeu G, Giovannini M. The fate of the brain cholinergic neurons in neurodegenerative diseases. Brain Res 2017;1670:173–84.

Petersson SD, Philippou E. Mediterranean Diet, cognitive function, and dementia: a systematic review of the evidence. Adv Nutr 2016;7:889–904.

Porsteinsson AP, Antonsdottir IM. An update on the advancements in the treatment of agitation in Alzheimer's disease. Esp Opin Pharmacother 2017;18(6):611–20.

Preuss UW, Wong JW, Koller G. Treatment of behavioral and psychological symptoms of dementia: a systematic review. Psychiatr Pol 2016;50(4):679–715.

Qosa H, Mohamed LA, Batarseh YS et al. Extra-virgin olive oil attenuates amyloid-β and tau pathologies in the brains of TgSwD1 mice. J Nutr Biochem 2015;26:1479–90.

Ransohoff RM. How neuroinflammation contributes to neurodegeneration. Science 2016;353(6301):777–83.

Rapp MA, Schnaider-Beeri M, Grossman HT et al. Increased hippocampal plaques and tangles in patients with Alzheimer disease with a lifetime history of major depression. Arch Gen Psychiatry 2006;63(2):161–7.

Raz L, Knoefel J, Bhaskar K. The neuropathology and cerebrovascular mechanisms of dementia. J Cereb Blood Flow Metab 2016;36:179–86.

Rigacci S. Olive oil phenols as promising multi-targeting agents against Alzheimer's disease. Adv Exp Med Biol 2015;863:1–20.

Ritter AR, Leger GC, Miller JB et al. Neuropsychological testing in pathologically verified Alzheimer's disease and frontotemporal dementia. Alzheimer Dis Assoc Disord 2017;31(3):187–91.

Roalf D, Moberg MJ, Turetsky BI et al. A quantitative meta-analysis of olfactory dysfunction in mild cognitive impairment. J Neurol Neurosurg Psychiatry 2017;88:226–32.

Rosenberg RN, Lambracht-Washington D, Yu G et al. Genomics of Alzheimer disease: a review. JAMA Neurol 2016;73(7):867–74.

Ruthirakuhan M, Herrmann N, Seuridjan I et al. Beyond immunotherapy: new approaches for disease modifying treatments for early Alzheimer's disease. Exp Opin Pharmacother 2016;17(18):2417–29.

Sabbagh MN, Schauble B, Anand K et al. Histopathology and florbetaben PET in patients incorrectly diagnosed with Alzheimer's disease. J Alzheimers Dis 2017;56(2):441–6.

Sachdeva A, Chandra M, Choudhary M et al. Alcohol-related dementia and neurocognitive impairment: a review study. Int J High Risk Behav Addict 2016;5(3):e27976.

Sadowsky CH, Galvin JE. Guidelines for the management of cognitive and behavioral problems in dementia. J Am Board Fam Med 2012;25(3):350–66.

Sarro L, Tosakulwong N, Schwarz CG et al. An investigation of cerebrovascular lesions in dementia with Lewy bodies compared to Alzheimer's disease. Alzheimers Dement 2017;13(3):257–66.

Scammel TE, Winrow CJ. Orexin receptors: pharmacology and therapeutic opportunities. Annu Rev Pharmacol Toxicol 2011;51:243–66.

Schellenberg GD, Montine TJ. The genetics and neuropathology of Alzheimer's disease. Acta Neuropatholo 2012;124(3):305–23.

Schott JM, Warren JD, Barhof F et al. Suspected early dementia. BMJ 2011;343:d5568.

Schroek JL, Ford J, Conway EL et al. Review of safety and efficacy of sleep medicines in older adults. Clin Therapeutics 2016;38(11):2340–72.

Schwartz M, Deczkowska A. Neurological disease as a failure of brain-immune crosstalk: the multiple faces of neuroinflammation. Trends Immonol 2016;37(10):668–79.

Sharma N, Singh AN. Exploring biomarkers for Alzheimer's disease. J Clin Diag Res 2016;10(7):KE01–06.

Siever LJ. Neurobiology of aggression and violence. Am J Psychiatry 2008;165:429–42.

Simonsen AH, Herukka SK, Andreasen N et al. Recommendations for CSF AD biomarkers in the diagnostic evaluation of dementia. Alzheimers Dement 2017;13(3):285–95.

Spies PE, Claasen JA, Peer PG et al. A prediction model to calculate probability of Alzheimer's disease using cerebrospinal fluid biomarkers. Alzheimers Dement 2013;9(3):262–8.

Spies PE, Verbeek MM, van Groen T et al. Reviewing reasons for the decreased CSF Abeta42 concentration in Alzheimer disease. Front Biosci (Landmark Ed) 2012;17:2024–34.

Spira AP, Gottesman RF. Sleep disturbance: an emerging opportunity for Alzheimer's disease prevention? Int Psychogeriatr 2017;29(4):529–31.

Stahl SM. Does treating hearing loss prevent or slow the progress of dementia? Hearing is not all in the ears, but who's listening? CNS Spectr 2017;22(3):247–50.

Stahl SM. Stahl's essential psychopharmacology: the prescriber's guide. 6th ed. New York, NY: Cambridge University Press; 2017b.

Stahl SM. Parkinson's disease psychosis as a serotonin-dopamine imbalance syndrome. CNS Spectr 2016;21(4):271–5.

Stahl SM. Mechanism of action of pimavanserin in Parkinson's disease psychosis: targeting serotonin 5HT2A and 5HT2C receptors. CNS Spectr 2016b;21(4):271–5.

Stahl SM. Stahl's essential psychopharmacology: neuroscientific basis and practical applications. 4th ed. New York, NY: Cambridge University Press; 2013.

Stahl SM, Morrissette DA. Stahl's illustrated sleep and wake disorders. New York, NY: Cambridge University Press; 2016.

Stahl SM, Morrissette DA. Stahl's illustrated violence: neural circuits, genetics, and treatment. New York, NY: Cambridge University Press; 2014.

Stahl SM, Morrissette DA, Cummings M et al. California State Hospital Violence Assessment and Treatment (Cal-VAT) guidelines. CNS Spectr 2014;19(5):449–65.

Takada LT, Kim MO, Cleveland RW et al. Genetic prion disease: experience of a rapidly progressive dementia center in the United States and a review of the literature. Am J Med Gen B Neuropsychiatr Genet 2017;174(1):36–69.

Tarawneh R, Holtzman DM. The clinical problem of symptomatic Alzheimer disease and mild cognitive impairment. Cold Spring Harbor Perspect Med 2012;2(5):a006148.

Tariot PN, Aisen PS. Can lithium or valproate untie tangles in Alzheimer's disease? J Clin Psychiatry 2009;70(6):919–21.

Thomas AJ, Attems J, Colloby SJ et al. Autopsy validation of 123I-FP-CIT dopaminergic neuroimaging for the diagnosis of DLB. Neurology 2017;88:1–8.

Thomas AJ, Taylor JP, McKeith I et al. Development of assessment toolkits for improving the diagnosis of Lewy body dementias: feasibility study within the DIAMOND Lewy study. Int J Geriatr Psychiatry 2017b;32(12):1280–1304.

Todd TW, Petrucelli L. Insights into the pathogenic mechanisms of Chromosome 9 open reading frame 72 (C9orf72) repeat expansions. J Neurochem 2016;138 (Suppl 1):145–62.

Togo T, Isojima D, Akatsu H et al. Clinical features of argyrophilic grain disease: a retrospective survey of cases with neuropsychiatric symptoms. Am J Geriatr Psychiatry 2005;13(12):1083–91.

Torrisi M, Cacciola A, Marra A et al. Inappropriate behaviors and hypersexuality in individuals with dementia; an overview of a neglected issue. Geriatr Gerontol Int 2017;17(6):865–74.

Tsai RM, Boxer AL. Therapy and clinical trials in frontotemporal dementia: past, present, and future. J Neurochem 2016;138(Suppl 1):211–21.

Tsuno N, Homma A. What is the association between depression and Alzheimer's disease? Exp Rev Neurother 2009;9(11):1667–76.

Tyebi S, Hannan AJ. Synaptopathic mechanisms of neurodegeneration and dementia: insights from Huntington's disease. Prog Neurobiol 2017;153:18–45.

Uzun S, Kozumplik O, Folnegovic-Smalc V. Alzheimer's dementia: current data review. Coll Antropol 2011;35(4):1333–7.

Van der Linde RM, Dening T, Stephan BC et al. Longitudinal course of behavioural and psychological symptoms of dementia: systematic review. Br J Psychiatry 2016;209:366–77.

van der Spek K, Gerritsen DL, Smallbrugge M et al. Only 10% of the psychotropic drug use for neuropsychiatric symptoms in patients with dementia is fully appropriate: The PROPER I-study. Int Psychogeriatr 2016;28(10):1589–95.

Venkataraman A, Kalk N, Sewell G et al. Alcohol and Alzheimer's disease — does alcohol dependence contribute to beta-amyloid deposition, neuroinflammation and neurodegeneration in Alzheimer's disease? Alcohol Alcoholism 2017;52(2):151–8.

Villemagne VL et al. Aβ-amyloid and tau imaging in dementia. Semin Nucl Med 2017;47:75–88.

Weintraub S, Wicklund AH, Salmon DP. The neuropsychological profile of Alzheimer disease. Cold Spring Harb Perspect Med 2012;2(4):a006171.

Weishaupt JH et al. Common molecular pathways in amyotrophic lateral sclerosis and frontotemporal dementia. Trends Mol Med 2016;22(9):769–83.

Wenning GK, Tison F, Seppi K et al. Development and validation of the Unified Multiple System Atrophy Rating Scale (UMSARS). Mov Disord 2004;19(12):1391–402.

Williams DR, Holton JL, Strand C et al. Pathological tau burden and distribution distinguishes progressive supranuclear palsy-parkinsonism from Richardson's syndrome. Brain 2007;130(Pt 6):1566–76.

Wimo A et al. The worldwide costs of dementia 2015 and comparisons with 2010. Alzheimers Dement 2017;13:1–7.

Wisniewski T, Drummond E. Developing therapeutic vaccines against Alzheimer's disease. Expert Rev Vaccines 2016;15(3):401–15.

Wuwongse S, Chang RC, Law AC. The putative neurodegenerative links between depression and Alzheimer's disease. Prog Neurobiol 2010;92(4):362–75.

Xu Y et al. Meta-analysis of risk factors for Parkinson's disease dementia. Transl Neurodegen 2016;5(11):1–8.

Yaffe K, Tocco M, Petersen RC et al. The epidemiology of Alzheimer's disease: laying the foundation for drug design, conduct, and analysis of clinical trials. Alzheimers Dement 2012;8(3):237–42.

Yan R. Stepping closer to treating Alzheimer's disease patients with BACE1 inhibitor drugs. Transl Neurodegen 2016;5:13.

Yang L, Yan J, Jin X et al. Screening for dementia in older adults: comparison of Mini-Mental State Examination, Min-Cog, Clock Drawing Test and AD8. PLOS ONE 2016;11(12):e0168949.

Yang T, Sun Y, Lu Z et al. The impact of cerebrovascular aging on vascular cognitive impairment and dementia. Ageing Res Rev 2017;34:15–29.

Yang W, Yu S. Synucleinopathies: common features and hippocampal manifestations. Cell Mol Life Sci 2017;74(8):8466–80.

Yeh HL, Tsai SJ. Lithium may be useful in the prevention of Alzheimer's disease in individuals at risk of presenile familial Alzheimer's disease. Med Hypotheses 2008;71(6):948–51.

Zhang Y, Cai J, An L et al. Does music therapy enhance behavioral and cognitive function in elderly dementia patients? A systematic review and meta-analysis. Ageing Res Rev 2017;35:1–11.

Zillox LA, Chadrasekaran K, Kwan JY et al. Diabetes and cognitive impairment. Curr Diab Rep 2016;16(87):1–11.

Stahl's Illustrated

Optional
Posttest and
CME Certificate

Release/Expiration Dates
Released: July, 2018
CME Credit Expires: June, 2021

Posttest Study Guide

This optional posttest with CME credits is available for a fee (waived for NEI Members).
NOTE: the posttest can only be submitted online. The below posttest questions have been
provided solely as a study tool to prepare for your online submission. **_Faxed/mailed_**
copies of the posttest cannot be processed and will be returned to the sender. If you do
not have access to a computer, contact customer service at +1-888-535-5600.

(Figures containing referenced information in parenthesis)

1. Marilyn is a 75-year-old patient who recently passed away following a 5-year battle
   with dementia. Autopsy reveals amyloid plaque pathology in various regions of
   Marilyn's brain, including neocortex and hippocampus, striatum, and brainstem with
   no involvement of the cerebellum. According to the Thal phases of amyloid pathology,
   Marilyn's amyloid pathology would be categorized as: *(Fig 1.3)*

   A. Phase 1   D. Phase 4
   B. Phase 2   E. Phase 5
   C. Phase 3

2. Martha is a 68-year-old patient with a family history of dementia. Genotyping of this
   patient reveals a mutation in her gene for amyloid precursor protein (APP). Which APP
   mutation is *not* associated with increased development of familial Alzheimer's disease?
   (Fig 1.16)

   A. Swedish mutation   D. London mutation
   B. Icelandic mutation   E. All of the above mutations
   C. Flemish mutation   are associated with increased
                                     development of familial
                                     Alzheimer's disease

---

3. Harold is a 63-year-old man enrolled in a clinical trial utilizing anti-amyloid immunotherapy for the treatment and/or prevention of Alzheimer's disease. Which of the following antibodies bind to fibrillar amyloid beta? *(Fig 1.62)*

A. Solanezumab   D. All of the above

B. Bapineuzumab   E. A and B only

C. Aducanumab   F. B and C only

4. Walter is a 61-year-old patient with alpha-synucleinopathy dementia with Lewy bodies. It is hypothesized that oligomerization and aggregation of pathological alpha-synuclein may stem from: *(Fig 2.4)*

A. Inflammatory particles   D. All of the above

B. Accumulation of pathological tau protein   E. None of the above

C. High levels of dopamine

5. Elizabeth is a 71-year-old patient with multiple system atrophy. Magnetic resonance imaging (MRI) of her brain would likely reveal which tell-tale sign? *(Fig 2.22)*

A. Hot cross buns   D. All of the above

B. Hummingbird   E. None of the above

C. Morning glory

6. Adele is a 75-year-old patient with behavioral variant frontotemporal dementia. Upon autopsy, it is revealed that this patient has no tau-positive pathology but an abundance of TAR-DNA binding protein 43 (TDP-43) pathology. TDP-43 pathology is associated with mutations in the gene for: *(Fig 3.3)*

A. Microtubule associated protein tau (MAPT)   C. Fused in sarcoma (FUS)

B. Chromosome 9 open reading frame 72 (C9orf72)

7. Marian is a 67-year-old patient with semantic variant primary progressive aphasia (svPPA). Neuropsychological tests of this patient would most likely show deficits in: *(Fig 3.17)*

A. Speech output   C. Word finding

B. Confrontational naming

8. Ellie is a 59-year-old patient who presents with hypoglycemia. She also presents with symptoms that could be either dementia or delirium. One key feature that can help differentiate delirium from dementia is: *(Fig 4.9)*

A. Memory deficits

B. Disorientation

C. Psychosis

D. Acute and fluctuating course

9. Joe is a 71-year-old man presenting with profound memory loss. He has a history of alcohol abuse, a brother with Alzheimer's disease, and complains of ophthalmoplegia. His most likely diagnosis is: *(Fig 4.11)*

A. Dementia with Lewy bodies

B. Wernicke–Korsakoff syndrome

C. Alzheimer's disease

D. Frontotemporal dementia

10. George is a 74-year-old patient diagnosed with Parkinson's disease 7 years ago. He has recently begun to show symptoms of psychosis, especially visual hallucinations. Which psychotropic agent is FDA-approved for the treatment of psychosis in Parkinson's disease? *(Fig 5.28)*

A. Quetiapine

B. Clozapine

C. Pimavanserin

D. Olanzapine

Instructions for Optional Online Posttest and CME Certificate
There is a fee for the optional posttest (waived for NEI Members).

1. Read the book

2. Complete the posttest and evaluation, available only online at **www.neiglobal.com/CME** (under "Book")

3. Print your certificate (if a score of 70% or more is achieved)

Questions? Call +1-888-535-5600, or email CustomerService@neiglobal.com

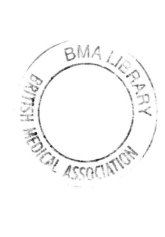